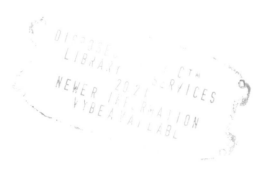

Practical Management of Asthma

Third Edition

Practical Management of Asthma

Third Edition

Tim Clark, MD, FRCP
Professor of Pulmonary Medicine, Imperial College School of Medicine
at the National Heart and Lung Institute
Consultant Physician, Royal Brompton Hospital

John Rees, MD, FRCP
Consultant Physician, Guy's Hospital
Senior Lecturer in Medicine, United Medical and Dental Schools of
Guy's and St Thomas's Hospitals

MARTIN DUNITZ

© Tim Clark and John Rees, 1985, 1996, 1998

First published in the United Kingdom in 1985
by Martin Dunitz Limited Ltd, The Livery House,
7–9 Pratt Street, London NW1 0AE

First edition 1985
Reprinted 1985
Reprinted 1986

Second edition 1996
Third edition 1998

A CIP catalogue record for this book is available from the British Library

ISBN 1-85317-587-0

Composition by Scribe Design, Gillingham, Kent, UK
Printed and bound in Singapore by Kyodo Printing Pte Ltd

Contents

Preface   vii
Introduction   ix

1   Making the diagnosis   1
2   Natural history of asthma   18
3   Precipitating factors in asthma   27
4   Management of acute asthma   46
5   Management of chronic asthma   62
6   Childhood asthma   80
7   Asthma in general practice   93
8   Inflammation and allergy   99
9   Methods of drug delivery   114
10   Physical and psychological treatments   140
11   Patient education   144

References   149
Useful addresses   156
Acknowledgements   157
Index   159

Preface

Since the first edition of this book more than a decade ago there have been many changes in asthma management. These have led to the development of asthma guidelines and consensus reports based on the proposition that airway inflammation plays an important and probably key role in asthma pathogenesis and there is now general agreement that chronic asthma is best treated by preventing airway inflammation. New information on the pathophysiology of the inflammatory process is leading to new possibilities in treatment such as modification of leukotriene function. There has also been an evolution in our standards of care so that control of asthma now demands patients achieving a normal quality of life with freedom from adverse effects of therapeutic interventions and restoration of lung function.

The acceleration of changes in asthma management strategy has led us to a further revision, in the hope that we can summarize these further changes that have taken place in a comprehensive but synoptic manner. Our aim is therefore once more to provide a concise and readable account of the management of this disorder for practising clinicians. The book is not a specialist treatise, but does include references for further reading as many clinicians find it helpful to supplement a practical manual with background information.

We hope this third edition will continue to provide practical advice about a common illness that leads to a very substantial socio-economic burden on individuals and society. The growth in prevalence, particularly in children, means that asthma is encountered frequently in general practice as well as in hospitals so we hope this practical manual will be of assistance to all those looking after asthma patients.

In many countries asthma care is also being carried out by health professionals other than doctors and we hope this book will be useful for them as well. Treatment protocols implemented by health professionals can enable asthma care to be improved in all countries throughout the world and the need for a practical guide is very important. This book has largely been written for European readers but we hope it can be of value in countries elsewhere in the world. Our main hope continues to be to improve the prospects for patients with asthma by clarifying for clinicians the issues concerning diagnosis and treatment and by drawing attention to the scope for effective pharmacological management. If this book can help a few patients to control their asthma successfully, then it will have been worthwhile.

T.J.H. Clark and P.J. Rees

Introduction

Asthma is a condition which has been known and described for more than 2,000 years. The word itself derives from a Greek word meaning panting. Over this period the seriousness with which it has been regarded has varied.[1] In the seventeenth century Thomas Willis was certainly aware of the seriousness of the condition and the difficulties of its treatment.[2] However, by the late nineteenth century the American physician and author Oliver Wendell Holmes was able to describe it as a 'slight ailment which prolongs longevity'.[1]

During the last twenty or thirty years there has been an increased understanding of the wide spectrum of the disease. Over the same period a number of effective, safe treatments have been developed. Little progress has been made in finding a cure for asthma in terms of removing the underlying reason for the airway narrowing, but in most cases it is possible to suppress the disease by pharmacological means without significant side-effects.

Despite these advances, the mortality from asthma remains depressingly constant. In Britain this is around 2,000 annually. In New Zealand a recent epidemic has settled but illustrates that modern medication by itself is insufficient to reduce mortality.[3] There is also a significant morbidity, producing loss of time from school and work and in some cases prolonged disability.

It seems that many of these problems stem from a failure to recognize the diagnosis of asthma and to use the available treatments appropriately. These persisting failures persuaded us that there was a need for a book dealing with the practical management of asthma. The sales of the first edition confirmed this view and we hope that revisions made in this second edition will also meet this need.

Asthma is a common condition affecting people of all ages (Fig. I.1). Most practitioners are involved in the management of some asthmatic patients and it is often a rewarding condition to treat. There is a great variation, though, in the severity of asthma and in the pattern of the problems it presents. Some patients have persistent airflow obstruction which, although it varies in severity, never leaves them free from wheezing. Most have a labile form of asthma in which they may be symptom-free most of the time. It is difficult to predict those whose lives may be at risk from sudden severe attacks of asthma.

Children with asthma are often given the label 'wheezy bronchitis' in the belief that this may spare parental anxiety associated with the word 'asthma'. The label that is given is of no great consequence as long as the children are treated appropriately. However,

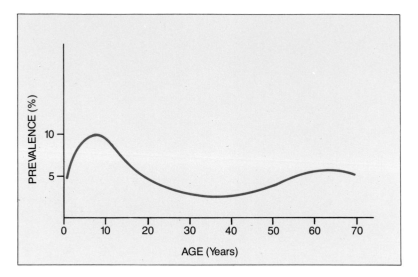

Figure I.1 Prevalence of asthma at various ages.

there is a tendency, once the diagnosis of wheezy bronchitis has been made, to use inappropriate treatment with antibiotics rather than treatment directed at the airflow obstruction itself.

The danger in older patients is that airflow obstruction will be dismissed as a consequence of cigarette smoking and therefore irreversible. The only way of being certain that reversible obstruction is not left untreated is formally to assess the responses to treatment in all such patients. This requires some objective assessment period, since there is no value in leaving patients with irreversible obstruction on treatments that are of no benefit.

WHAT IS ASTHMA?

The predominant clinical features of asthma are breathlessness and wheezing, which are easily recognized, but there have been many disputes about the definition of asthma. The NIH International Consensus Report on the diagnosis and management of asthma defined asthma as follows:[4]

> Asthma is a chronic inflammatory disorder of the airways in which many cells play a role, including mast cells and eosinophils. In susceptible individuals this inflammation causes symptoms which are usually associated with widespread but variable airflow obstruction that is often reversible either spontaneously or with treatment, and causes an associated increase in airway responsiveness to a variety of stimuli.

This emphasizes the central role of airway inflammation and variability of airflow obstruction which both help determine the appropriate therapeutic response.

THE SCALE OF THE PROBLEM

Even fairly precise definitions are subject to local interpretation in different countries and this means that any geographical variations in respiratory disease rates must be interpreted cautiously. Furthermore, it is difficult to be sure of the true prevalence of asthma because of the difficulties in definition and diagnosis. Nevertheless there are some marked differences in the prevalence of asthma which have been reasonably well established.[5]

In Britain or the United States a questionnaire on respiratory symptoms will usually produce a positive response rate of 20–30 per cent to a question on the prevalence of wheezing. Many of these subjects would not fit into a conventional diagnosis of asthma, and in these countries the actual prevalence of asthma is nearer 5 per cent. Australia and New Zealand have higher rates while those in China are lower, more like 2 per cent.

Some communities have more extreme differences in the prevalence of asthma. Rural communities in New Guinea and Gambia, and Eskimos have very low rates. The classic example of a community with a high prevalence of asthma is the isolated Atlantic island of Tristan da Cunha, where the prevalence rate is over 30 per cent. The high rate has been traced to three asthmatic women among the original fifteen settlers on the island.[6] While this demonstrates the influence of genetic factors in asthma, other evidence from the movement of communities from rural to urban districts shows the importance of environmental factors, because migration to more affluent and industrialized locations is associated with increases in prevalence. Such increases are also seen over time in most countries, suggesting that increased environmental hazards promote the spread of asthma. If the environmental causes for this can be established, appropriate environmental control measures might be effective.

A general practice population of 2,500 will contain at least 125 patients with asthma. These patients will have a wide range of severity, age of onset and different treatment requirements. There is the opportunity and the obligation for all practitioners to develop their expertise in the diagnosis and treatment of asthma. Perhaps then the morbidity and mortality from asthma will at last begin to decline. If our book helps to contribute to this decline, we shall be well satisfied.

1
Making the diagnosis

BACKGROUND

The clinical features of asthma are breathlessness and wheezing. Typical young asthmatic patients are easy to recognize. However, the clinical presentation is by no means uniform, reflecting the many factors involved in the development and course of asthma. The definition of asthma we gave in the introduction indicates that symptoms are often episodic and triggered by various factors. The inflammatory nature of asthma accounts for features such as cough and sputum and for the diagnostic overlap with chronic bronchitis. Thus, although many patients have episodic symptoms and known triggers punctuating periods without symptoms, many other patients present a different picture.

PROBLEMS IN DIAGNOSIS

Patients with asthma do not always complain of intermittent wheezing and certain presentations may mask the diagnosis of asthma.

Cough

Particularly in children, a cough may be the only presenting symptom of asthma.[7] This is likely to be most troublesome at night. In such circumstances it is usually possible to show variation in airflow obstruction from regular peak flow recordings or provocation of bronchoconstriction on exercise testing (see pages 13 and 15).

Irreversible airflow obstruction

In older patients the problem arises of differentiating between asthma and chronic bronchitis with or without emphysema. This is best approached from a therapeutic standpoint. If airflow obstruction is present then, whatever you choose to call it, what matters is how much improvement can be produced by treatment. Therefore, the management of all patients with symptomatic airflow obstruction should start with attempts to reverse the obstruction, monitoring the results with peak flow readings if possible.

This approach will bring to light asthmatic patients who initially seem to have persistent airflow obstruction but who improve markedly on treatment, and it will also establish whether such treatment will be worthwhile in those with chronic airflow obstruction.

Paroxysmal nocturnal dyspnoea

Repeated nocturnal waking with shortness of breath is most often a symptom of left heart failure, once known as 'cardiac asthma'. However, asthma itself is typically at its worst in the early hours of the morning. In some patients, where heart disease and respiratory disease occur together, differentiating the cause of nocturnal breathlessness can be difficult and often requires a trial of appropriate therapy.

Cor pulmonale

Very occasionally, persistent airflow obstruction in asthma produces right heart failure and some patients even present in this way when the diagnosis of asthma has not been made previously.[8] It may be that this is particularly likely to occur in patients with a reduced response in the respiratory centre to blood gas changes.

Asthma in children

Attacks of wheezing are very common in infants under one year of age. Over one-third of such infants go on to have asthma later in childhood.

Differential diagnosis of asthma

Condition	Diagnostic points
1. Chronic irreversible airflow obstruction	• Only accept after failure of vigorous attempts at reversal of obstruction
2. Upper airway obstruction	• Usually persistent • Inspiratory stridor often evident on examination (Fig. 1.2) • Typical findings on flow–volume loop (Fig. 1.1b)
3. Pulmonary oedema	• May be characteristic findings on ECG, chest X-ray and examination
4. Recurrent respiratory infections	• Airflow obstruction absent • Negative exercise test • No significant diurnal variation of peak flow

---

There has been a tendency to diagnose repeated attacks of wheezing in early childhood as being 'wheezy bronchitis' because it is felt that this will produce less anxiety among parents than a label of asthma. This is often associated with inadequate or inappropriate treatment.

The diagnosis of asthma does not cause parents unnecessary worry if it is accompanied by sufficient explanation of its likely course and management. Good control of asthma requires active participation on the part of the patient or parent, and this is likely to occur only if they are kept suitably informed.

AETIOLOGY

It has been common practice to divide asthma into extrinsic and intrinsic forms. There is a degree of overlap, and many asthmatics, particularly adults, do not fall clearly into either group and the usefulness of this distinction is questioned.

Extrinsic asthma

This has identifiable external triggering factors, such as specific allergens. It is common in young people and is associated with positive immediate skin-prick tests and a personal or family history of asthma, hay fever and eczema.

Intrinsic asthma

This is more common in older patients. There are no obvious triggering stimuli other than respiratory infections and, often, there is less reversibility, with more long-standing airflow obstruction of some degree.

Characteristic features of extrinsic and intrinsic asthma

Most asthmatics fall broadly into the groups below. There is, however, overlap between the two.

Extrinsic	Intrinsic
• Starts in childhood	• Often starts in adulthood
• Eczema and rhinitis often present	• Often persistent symptoms
• Positive skin tests to common allergens	• Negative skin tests
• Precipitating factors evident from history	• No obvious precipitating factor, except infection
• Episodic	• Aspirin-sensitive subjects usually intrinsic
• Positive family history	

The flow volume loop is obtained by asking the patient to inspire to total lung capacity, then measuring flow continuously as he or she expires as fast as possible to residual volume and then inspires again to total lung capacity. The normal flow volume loop and the flow volume loop in asthma are compared in Fig. 1.1a. The large airway obstructions shown in Figs 1.1b–d can clinically mimic asthma but are easily detected by the typical picture in the flow volume loop.

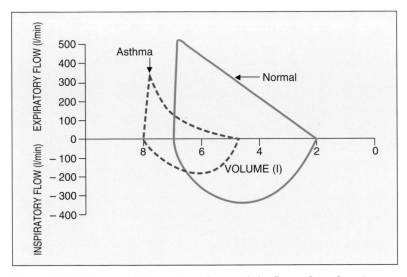

Figure 1.1 (a) The normal flow volume loop and the flow volume loop in asthma showing overinflation and generalized airflow obstruction.

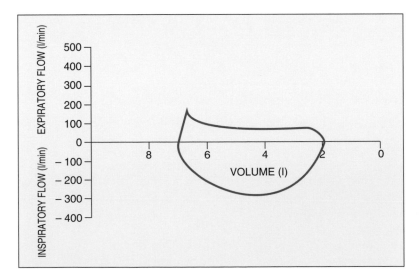

Figure 1.1 (b) A flow volume loop showing a flat expiratory limb. This picture is seen with obstruction in a single large intrathoracic airway, such as the lower trachea, susceptible to pressure changes.

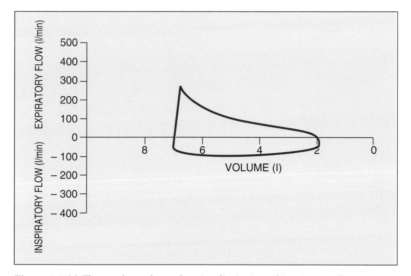

Figure 1.1 (c) Flow volume loop showing limitation of inspiratory flow consistent with a variable obstruction in a large extrathoracic airway. This would occur with a laryngeal lesion or a floppy segment in the upper trachea.

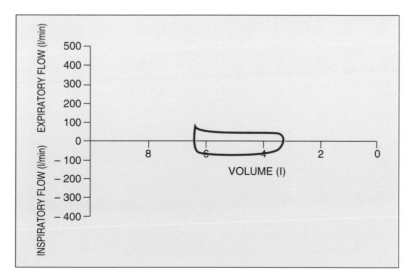

Figure 1.1 (d) Flow volume loop showing severe airflow limitation in expiration and inspiration. This picture is seen with rigid obstructions in a large airway, a neoplasm of the trachea, for example.

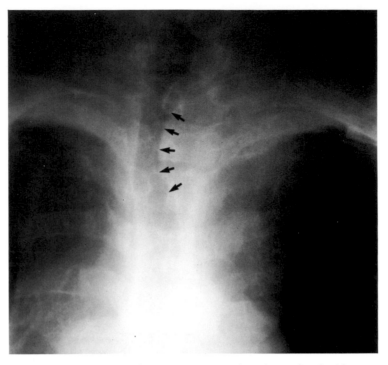

Figure 1.2 Large airway obstruction can sometimes be confused with asthma. This X-ray shows an upper mediastinal tumour which is compressing the trachea (see arrows) producing shortness of breath and an inspiratory monophonic wheeze.

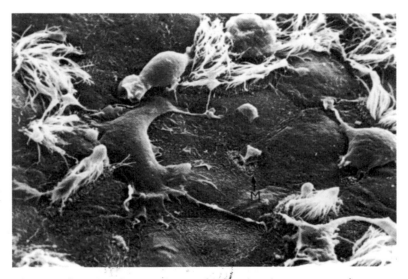

Figure 1.3 Scanning electron micrograph of bovine airway mucosa after rhinovirus infection, showing loss of cilia and presence of macrophages. Such disruption may explain the temporary increase in airway reactivity after viral infections.

Bronchial hyperresponsiveness

In all types of asthma an underlying problem seems to lie in an abnormal reactivity of the airways; that is, they narrow excessively in response to stimuli which would not affect normal subjects. Subjects with hay fever form an intermediate group between normals and asthmatics. Even healthy subjects may show an increase in the 'twitchiness' or responsiveness of their airways to nonspecific stimuli for up to six weeks after viral upper respiratory tract infections (Fig. 1.3).[9] This temporary increase in reactivity occurs because such infections denude the tracheal and bronchial mucosa, exposing sensory receptors in the mucosa. However, neurological reflexes are only a part of the story of the responsiveness of the airways. Airway inflammation is likely to be the main cause of airway hyperresponsiveness.

Many stimuli to airway responsiveness are nonspecific and may act either by directly stimulating airway smooth muscle (e.g. histamine) or indirectly by the release of pharmacologically active mediators (e.g. exercise).

Specific mediator release

Immunological stimuli probably act by releasing active substances from mast cells. Allergens interact with specific IgE molecules on the walls of mast cells to release preformed mediators such as eosinophil chemotactic factor, neutrophil chemotactic factor and histamine. This initial mediator release results in the production of other mediators such as prostaglandins and leukotrienes by metabolism of arachidonic acid (see pages 100–2).

Although research workers have tended to keep the two factors (reflex nervous contraction and mediator release) separate it seems likely that the two are closely interrelated in clinical exacerbations of asthma.

Provoking factors

Those of importance in asthma are:

- Infections
- Inhaled allergens
- Dusts, environmental pollution
- Exercise
- Drugs
- Foods
- Occupations
- Psychological
- Hormonal
- Gastro-oesophageal reflux

These are dealt with in detail in Chapter 3.

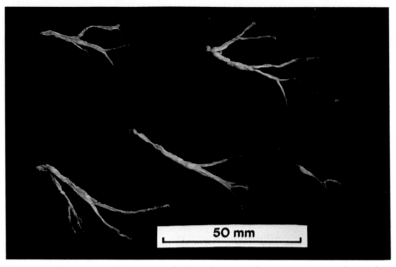

Figure 1.4 These viscid plugs coughed up by an asthmatic patient in the early hours of the morning were teased out to reveal casts of the airways.

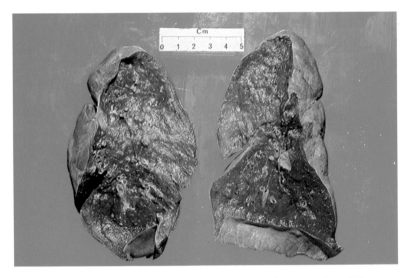

Figure 1.5 The lungs of a 14-year-old girl who died of acute asthma. The bronchial walls are thickened and obstructed by tenacious mucus plugs.

PATHOLOGICAL CHANGES IN ASTHMA

The three main factors producing airflow obstruction in asthma are:[10]

- Retention of bronchial secretions
- Thickening of the bronchial wall
- Bronchoconstriction

Mucus plugging

The lungs in fatal cases of asthma are overinflated. They fail to collapse when the chest is opened because of widespread mucus plugging of the airways. Such plugs, made up of yellow viscid mucus and desquamated epithelial cells, are often coughed up during acute attacks (Fig. 1.4). This sometimes produces marked relief of symptoms. The mucus in asthma is abnormally sticky and also has in inhibitory action on the cilia in the airways, both factors predisposing to mucus retention and plugging (Fig. 1.5).

Changes in the bronchial wall

The bronchial wall in asthma is also abnormal.[10] Inflammatory cells, particularly eosinophils, invade the wall, which becomes oedematous. Between exacerbations these changes are reversible but in the longer term bronchial mucous glands may enlarge and the bronchial smooth muscles and the collagen beneath the basement membrane may become thickened (Fig. 1.6). There may be an increase in the collagen laid down beneath the basement membrane producing sub-basement membrane fibrosis. This may produce a remodelling of the airways with irreversible obstruction.

Airflow obstruction

This, of course, is the main physiological finding in asthma.

Measuring respiratory function   This is simple to quantify with inexpensive portable equipment. Various portable peak flow meters are available for home recording (Fig. 1.7) and compare well with the standard meter (Fig. 1.8). Although more complex tests may

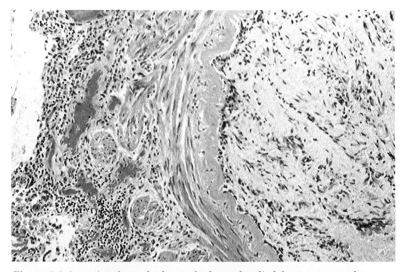

Figure 1.6 A section from the lung of a boy who died from severe asthma. The bronchial lumen on the right is blocked by a mucus plug. The basement membrane is thickened and the smooth muscle is hypertrophied.

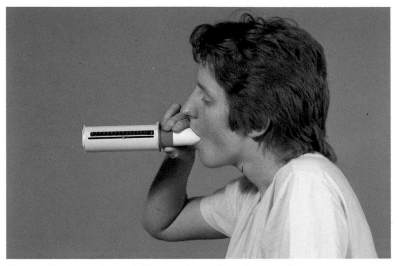

Figure 1.7 Being light, portable and cheap, the mini peak flow meter is suitable for home monitoring.

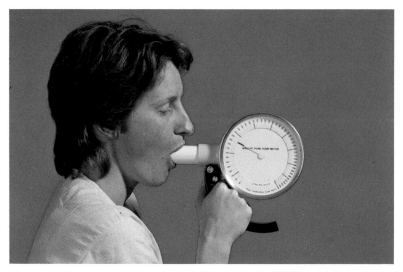

Figure 1.8 The standard Wright's peak flow meter is widely used. It is more robust than the mini peak flow meter shown above but much more expensive.

show overinflation and various other features of airflow obstruction, they add little to measurements of peak expiratory flow rate. There is a good deal more benefit to be obtained from frequently repeated simple tests of respiratory function at home than by occasional visits for elaborate testing at lung function laboratories.

Asthma is by definition a variable disease and the treatment is often adjusted to the severity. About 20 per cent of asthmatic patients have a very poor perception of moderate

MAY	MAXIMUM PEAK FLOW			COMMENTS
	MORN	AFTER-NOON	EVE	
1	310	360	345	
2	300	345	345	
3	300	355	360	
4	280	340	330	
5	275	345	335	
6	235	265	245	Woke at night wheezy
7	230	245	245	10 extra puffs of salbutamol
8	185	245	230	started prednisolone 40mg
9	210	240	235	pred 40mg
10	235	260	270	pred 40mg
11	275	325	310	,,
12	310	370	355	,,

Figure 1.9 A diary card of peak flow measurements and other comments. The peak flow is the maximum of three measurements taken before any inhaler use first thing in the morning, in the afternoon and last thing at night. In the comments section the patient can record inhaler use or other symptoms.

changes in the state of their asthma,[11] and in these patients peak flow monitoring is particularly important. They themselves may be unaware of a steady deterioration in their condition until acute severe asthma develops. Recording of peak flow in the management of asthma may be looked on as equivalent to urine testing in the management of diabetes mellitus.

How it is done   The peak flow meter is used by taking a full inspiration, putting the lips firmly around the mouthpiece with no leaks and producing a fast sharp expiration. This does not need to be continued to residual volume since the peak flow (maximum flow maintained for 10 msec) will occur right at the start of expiration. The best of three readings should be recorded. In asthma there is often a decrease in peak flow with repeated measurements.

Home peak flow measurement can be used for diagnosis as well as for monitoring treatment. Most patients can be taught to keep simple records of their readings on diary cards (Fig. 1.9). The peak flow should be recorded on the cards at the same time each day. These times should be early morning, late evening and also mid-afternoon if possible. Recordings

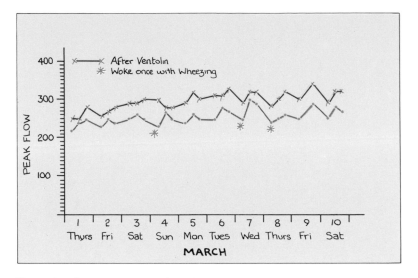

Figure 1.10 Some patients produce detailed technicolour charts of their peak flow results.

should be made before the use of any bronchodilator aerosols. Further measurements should be made at times of increased wheezing, for example if the patient is woken from sleep by asthma.

Many patients take great pride in producing beautiful colour charts of their recordings (Fig. 1.10). Such charts will often show the typical diurnal variation of airflow obstruction in asthma, with so called 'morning dipping' of peak flow by at least 15 per cent from evening values. The lowest point in the drop usually occurs between 2 am and 4 am, a time when many patients wake up breathless and asthmatic deaths more frequently occur. Portable peak flow meters with linear scales may not accurately measure flow throughout the range. Adjusted scales are available. When a patient becomes used to the readings of their own peak flow meter these inaccuracies may not be very important, but affect comparisons between machines.

Many acute exacerbations of asthma are preceded by periods of deteriorating control (Fig. 1.11). With a peak flow record these trends can easily be identified and appropriate action taken to prevent acute attacks. This is particularly important in those patients with poor perception of bronchoconstriction.[12] It is much better to anticipate exacerbations in this way rather than deal with them when they arise.

MAKING THE DIAGNOSIS

In typical cases the diagnosis of asthma will be obvious from the clinical history. Tests such as immediate skin prick tests only establish the existence of the atopic state, and do not help in the diagnosis of asthma (see Chapter 8). Establishing the diagnosis objectively relies on demonstrating variability of the airflow obstruction. There are a number of ways of doing this.

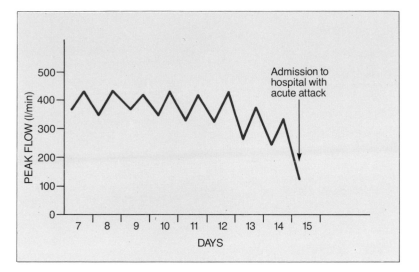

Figure 1.11 Home recordings of peak flow will often show gradual deterioration before the onset of an acute exacerbation. Suitable intervention at this point will often prevent the attack.

Reversibility with bronchodilators

The simplest way to confirm the diagnosis of asthma is to show improvement (15 per cent increase is usually taken as the criterion) in peak flow or forced expiratory volume in one second (FEV_1) twenty minutes after two puffs (200 mcg) of salbutamol or some other beta$_2$ agonist. Such changes do not occur in normal patients. In asthmatics this is likely to be successful only if the initial recordings are significantly below the predicted normal ranges (Figs. 1.12 and 1.13).

Diurnal variation

Recordings of peak flow for a week at home will often make the diagnosis obvious.[13] The criterion is a 15 per cent mean difference between the peak flow early in the morning and that in the evening. Patients can use a diary card as described previously, or simply make a table of peak flow on rising in the morning and on going to bed in the evening.

Exercise testing

If the lung function is normal when the patient is seen then it is possible to make a diagnosis by showing that the airways are abnormally reactive to stimuli which have little or no effect on normal people. Perhaps the simplest challenge test is to see the effect of six minutes vigorous exercise. In over 80 per cent of asthmatics peak flow will fall by at least 15 per cent after exercise (Fig. 1.14). The decline in peak flow may start during

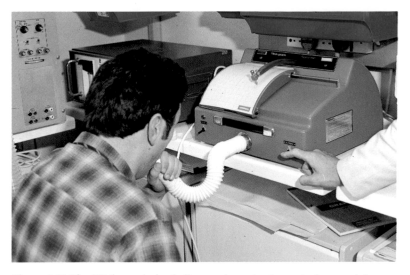

Figure 1.12 The Vitalograph dry bellows spirometer is most often used for measuring FEV_1 and forced vital capacity (FVC). In chronic airflow obstruction reversibility may be detectable in FVC or relaxed VC but not shown in peak flow recordings.

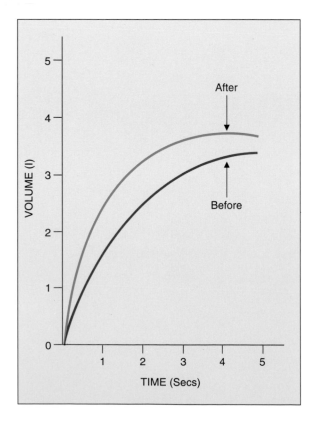

Figure 1.13 Spirometer tracing taken before and twenty minutes after a beta₂ agonist showing the typical reversibility of asthma.

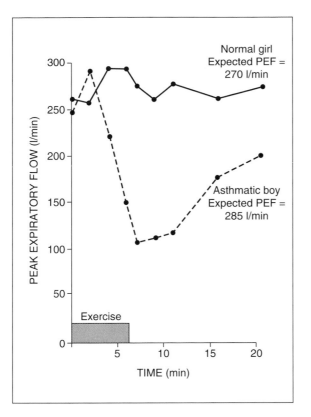

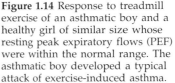

Figure 1.14 Response to treadmill exercise of an asthmatic boy and a healthy girl of similar size whose resting peak expiratory flows (PEF) were within the normal range. The asthmatic boy developed a typical attack of exercise-induced asthma.

exercise or there may be a temporary bronchodilatation during exercise itself, followed by a fall a few minutes later. Normal subjects usually show a slight increase in peak flow during exercise, possibly because of reduction in vagal tone.

A major part of the exercise stimulus seems to be drying and cooling of the airways related to increased ventilation.[14] Some laboratories have therefore replaced the exercise test with a period of hyperventilation breathing cold, dry air at rest. The results are very much the same and may also be mimicked by breathing ultrasonically nebulized distilled water. However, the apparatus is complicated and the simple method is for patients to exercise vigorously for five or six minutes, either by running around outside or up and down stairs. Peak flow should be recorded each minute after exercise for ten to fifteen minutes. As soon as the diagnostic criterion of a 15 per cent fall in peak flow has been reached, the bronchoconstriction should be reversed by inhalation of a beta$_2$ agonist. Such exercise provocation tests are perfectly safe in asthmatics in the absence of ischaemic heart disease.

Steroid trial

If there is evidence of airflow obstruction and it is not improved by inhaled beta$_2$ agonists then a trial of corticosteroids should be considered.[15] This is best done by establishing baseline peak flow rates by a week's home recording twice daily before therapy (Fig. 1.15). Oral prednisolone is then given at a dose of 30–40 mg once daily for two weeks

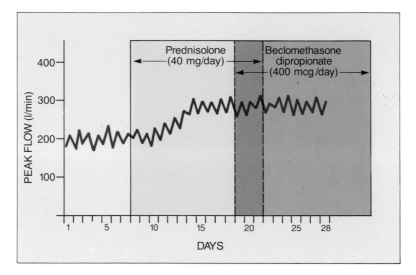

Figure 1.15 A trial of corticosteroids in stable airflow obstruction should have a control 'run-in' period followed by two weeks treatment at a dose of 30-40 mg per day. If there has been a satisfactory response, continued treatment with an inhaled steroid may be advisable.

while continuing beta$_2$ agonists as necessary. If there is going to be a response it will usually occur during this time.

The course of oral prednisolone is used purely to establish the diagnosis and does not commit the patient to further oral steroid therapy. The common practice is to switch from oral prednisolone to an inhaled steroid at the end of the test period, hoping that the improvement is then maintained on the inhaled drug.

Challenge testing

Some workers like to demonstrate the increased reactivity of the airways by challenging the airways with inhaled histamine or methacholine (Fig. 1.16).[16] Asthmatics bronchoconstrict at concentrations which have no effect on normal subjects. These challenge tests should only be performed in experienced laboratories and are not necessary in the vast majority of patients.

Even more problems occur during challenge testing with specific allergens. The problems come from difficulties in purification and standardization of the antigenic material, and from late asthmatic reactions six to twelve hours after challenge. The late reactions mean that patients must be kept under close observation for many hours after challenge and there must be facilities available for hospital admission. Such challenge testing is not necessary for diagnosis but may be important in occupational asthma and before considering desensitization (see Chapters 3 and 8).

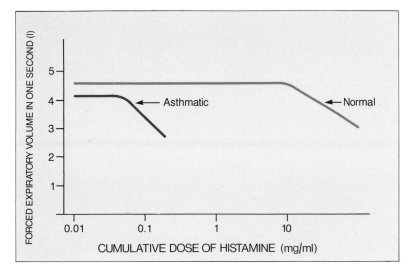

Figure 1.16 Asthmatics exposed to increasing doses of histamine or methacholine show airway narrowing at much lower doses than normal subjects. Subjects with atopic conditions but without asthma tend to form an intermediate group.

PRACTICAL POINTS

- The diagnosis of asthma relies on the demonstration of a variable degree of airflow obstruction. In patients who have airflow obstruction when they are examined, this can be detected by seeing the effects of inhaled bronchodilators or, if this fails, a short course of oral corticosteroids.
- When no airflow obstruction is present at the time of examination, but the story is suggestive of asthma, two simple methods are available.
  1. Diurnal variation may be detected by home peak flow recording.
  2. The effect on peak flow of a short bout of vigorous exercise can be assessed.
- Remember to consider asthma in patients who present with a cough, especially if this is mainly at night. Always listen to the patient's story carefully. Airflow obstruction is likely to be much more prominent and distressing in the early hours of the morning than later on in the surgery. When in doubt, give a trial of asthma treatment.
- In circumstances where objective measures of airflow are unavailable, diagnosis can usually be made from the symptoms.

2
Natural history of asthma

AGE OF PRESENTATION

Most new cases of asthma present in childhood or middle age. The relative proportions of patients presenting in the two main age groups vary between countries. Studies of the occurrence of asthma often use the term 'point prevalence' to indicate how many subjects have active asthma at the time. For this purpose active asthma means at least one attack or asthmatic treatment over the previous year.

The point prevalence varies from country to country but a reasonable global average is about 5%. In addition it varies with age; studies in children produce prevalence rates of 10–20%. Up to ten years of age new cases are frequent and remissions are also common. However, few new cases present in the late teens and twenties and the point prevalence drops. Over forty years of age the prevalence increases again. The incidence of new cases is less than in childhood but the asthma is more persistent and remissions less frequent.

A practitioner with a list of 2,500 patients can expect to have at least 125 patients with asthma. Many of these may have mild symptoms which have not been recognized as asthma.

SEX DIFFERENCES

Boys are more likely than girls to develop asthma by a ratio of about three to two. By adulthood, asthma has the same prevalence in both sexes, reflecting the fact that girls are less likely to lose their asthma during adolescence. Attacks of shortness of breath and wheezing occur with the same frequency in adult males and females. However, there has been a tendency for females to be diagnosed as asthmatic while males may be wrongly labelled with chronic airflow obstruction or chronic bronchitis and emphysema related to cigarette smoking.

THE OUTLOOK FOR CHILDHOOD ASTHMA

Parents are often reassured that their children will grow out of their asthma. Fortunately for many of them this is true, and there are a number of features which help to predict which children will improve and which will have continuing problems (Fig. 2.1). This

323 Children aged 7 with wheeze			
Free of wheeze for 3 years	Free of wheeze for 3 months to 3 years	Wheeze < once a week	Wheeze > once a week
Aged 21 33%	21%	26%	21%
Aged 28 33%	21%	22%	25%

Figure 2.1 The prognosis is worse for those with more severe, persistent asthma in childhood. Overall, there was a tendency to worsen between the ages of 21 and 28 in this study.[17]

broadly reassuring outlook is no reason not to treat all cases of childhood asthma vigorously. There is every reason to hope that good early treatment reduces respiratory problems later in life.

Children with infrequent episodes of wheezing and no persistent symptoms in their early years will be free of any problems with asthma by the age of twenty-one in more than 50 per cent of cases. Seventy per cent of those who have frequent, troublesome wheezing in childhood will continue to have asthma at the age of twenty-one, although about 70 per cent of these will have shown some improvement. Future problems can often be predicted from a severe onset of the asthma with frequent troublesome attacks during the first year of the disease.[17]

Other factors associated with a poorer prognosis are persistent airflow obstruction and associated atopic diseases in the patient or the family. Although there is some disagreement, onset below the age of three years is usually regarded as being more troublesome than onset later in childhood.

One year's freedom from trouble with asthma is no guarantee of lifelong freedom. A third of the children who have a year's remission are likely to have a recurrence of their asthma more than ten years later because the reactivity of their airways remains greater than normal. Airway reactivity can be reduced by removal from exposure to appropriate allergens (see Chapter 3) or by suitable prophylactic treatment (see Chapter 6). Although there is no evidence from long-term studies to confirm this belief it seems hopeful that such measures to reduce the 'twitchiness' and reactivity of the airways will reduce subsequent problems from asthma and make sustained remission more likely.

THE OUTLOOK FOR ADULT ASTHMA

Remission is much less likely to occur in adult asthmatics than in children. Many of these patients will have persistent airflow obstruction between exacerbations. They are less likely to show the typical childhood pattern of acute attacks punctuating periods of normality.

Adult asthmatics are more likely to be intrinsic (see page 3) and in older patients it is unusual to be able to identify an important external agent which precipitates their asthma (see Chapter 3).

MORBIDITY FROM ASTHMA

Asthma accounts for more absences from school than any other chronic disease. Studies demonstrating the underdiagnosis and undertreatment of childhood asthma[18,19] show that such figures are likely to be an underestimate of the total number of days lost through asthma. There are three main factors to consider in the morbidity of asthma: asthma itself, overprotection and treatment.

Asthma itself

The vast majority of asthmatic children treated appropriately with inhaled anti-inflammatory medication and bronchodilators will lose few days from school. Problems are likely to be much greater in those children whose asthma is unrecognized or is treated as bronchitis with antibiotics or antitussives. These children often lose a lot of time from school with so-called 'recurrent bronchitis' before the correct diagnosis is made.

Asthma in childhood can lead to problems with growth and chest deformity but these are very uncommon unless there is unremitting severe disease.

In adult asthmatics the more persistent symptoms may produce a significant disability and impose limitations on both occupational and social life.

Overprotection

Adequate education by the doctor should aim to avoid problems associated with parents being overprotective towards their asthmatic child. Virtually all asthmatic children can attend normal schools and, given appropriate treatment, take part in the majority of sporting activities there.

Behavioural disturbances arise in some asthmatic children but they are usually associated with severe, continuous asthma where both the disease and the parental reaction are likely to play a part. Such disturbances are difficult to define and quantify but aggressive behaviour and anxiety are more common in severe asthma. There is, however, no increase in enuresis, stammering or nervous tics.[20] Behavioral disturbances are best approached by building up the confidence of the parents and patients and by educating them to help in controlling the asthma. They need to know precisely what to do in acute exacerbations, and how they can reliably obtain further advice and help.

Treatment

Side-effects of individual drugs are dealt with later in the book. In general, the various treatments given for asthma have few significant side-effects, particularly if given by inhalation, and they are unlikely to contribute to any persisting morbidity. The one exception to this is oral corticosteroids. It is unusual to use long-term oral corticosteroids unless there are great problems with asthma control. In such cases the usual side-effects of corticosteroid treatment are to be expected (see table below), although they may be decreased by alternate-day use and minimization of the dose by the use of inhaled steroids (see Chapter 9). The suggestion that the risk of osteoporosis and fractures are minimal for asthmatics on corticosteroids has been shown to be untrue.[21] Patients on long-term steroids or with frequent courses (more than eight per year) are at considerable risk from such problems.

Of the other asthma treatments, adverse side-effects are most commonly seen with theophyllines, even with conventional doses and therapeutic drug levels (see page 53).

Side-effects of oral and parenteral corticosteroids

- Growth retardation in children
- Truncal obesity
- Hypertension
- Osteoporosis
- Aseptic bone necrosis
- Proximal myopathy
- Cataracts
- Poor wound healing
- Immunosuppression
- Amenorrhoea
- Hyperglycaemia
- Hyperlipidaemia
- Hypokalaemia
- Mood change
- Steroid psychosis
- Haemorrhage from peptic ulcers

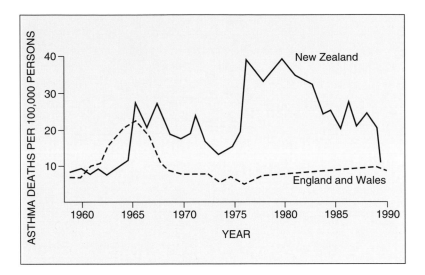

Figure 2.2 Asthma mortality in five- to thirty-four-year-olds in England and Wales and New Zealand during 1959–90.

Socio-economic aspects

Asthma is a major burden on the individual patient and society. It affects the quality of life and may impair schooling and work. Its costs are high: a recent study showed asthma costing $6.2 billion per annum in the USA with major expenditure on in-patient care and other direct medical costs. Cost-effective studies show that the costs of medication can be repaid by reducing both direct and indirect costs and especially by achieving a saving in in-patient admissions.

MORTALITY FROM ASTHMA

In the early part of this century the prevailing opinion was that deaths from asthma did not occur and that the presence of asthma was associated with longevity. This view had changed long before the increase in asthma deaths which occurred in a number of countries during the 1960s. This increase was contemporaneous with the use of high-strength isoprenaline inhalers. Originally this was attributed to the cardiac stimulatory effects of isoprenaline. However, it may well have happened because patients, having at last found a rapidly effective treatment, persisted with it in acute severe asthma when the effectiveness diminished and further help should have been sought. These patients in effect died of their asthma, the severity of which was partially masked by the inhaler. Lack of appropriate steroid treatment was probably more important than overuse of the aerosols, which merely indicated severity of asthma.

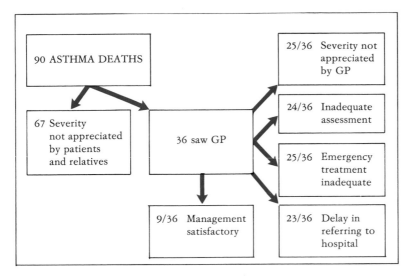

Figure 2.3 In 1982 the British Thoracic Association published its findings on ninety asthma deaths. A panel assessed the factors involved in the deaths and found deficiencies in assessment of severity and treatment in the majority of cases.

Since this temporary increase in mortality in the 1960s the death rate from asthma has shown a slow rise to around 2,000 deaths per year in England and Wales (Fig. 2.2). A further epidemic occurred in New Zealand in the late 1970s which was also associated with increased use of bronchodilators.[3,22] Subsequent studies in New Zealand and Canada could not establish whether this association was causal or simply an indicator of severity. A meta-analysis in 1993[23] has cast doubt on the association between beta$_2$ agonists and asthma deaths. Other studies have shown undertreatment and failure in access to care as important factors. For example, the 1982 British Thoracic Association study investigating asthma deaths found that, in the majority, undertreatment and inadequate appreciation of the severity of asthma by patients and doctors were much more likely to be involved than any potential harmful effect of treatment (Fig. 2.3).[24]

Preventive measures

A few deaths occur with very rapidly worsening asthma from a normal baseline.[24] Such catastrophic attacks are obviously difficult to treat in time but they are in the minority, and acute severe attacks usually occur from a background of worsening control. It is by stepping in with suitable treatment at this stage that we can hope to prevent mortality from asthma.

Most asthmatics will notice such a decline in control either from their symptoms or from increasing use and decreasing effect of their bronchodilator aerosols. This can be confirmed by peak flow readings. About 15 to 20 per cent of asthmatics do not notice moderate changes in their airflow obstruction.[11] They can, therefore, quietly deteriorate

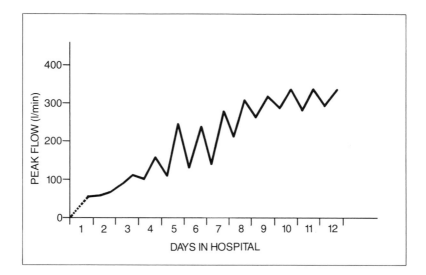

Figure 2.4 Peak flow rates taken at 6 am and 10 pm each day during recovery from a severe exacerbation of asthma. Patients often develop this marked diurnal variation of peak flow rate during recovery. They may be particularly vulnerable during this period and intensive treatment and supervision should be continued.

until they suddenly present with severe asthma.[12] For these patients regular home monitoring with a peak flow monitor is essential.

When patients are at risk

There appear to be periods of particular risk. These occur shortly after hospital discharge or, within hospital, after a move from an intensive care to a general ward during recovery from acute severe attacks. At such a time, diurnal variation is often particularly great and acute problems usually occur in the early hours of the morning.[25] The vigorous treatment given for the acute attack is meanwhile being reduced.

These problems are best avoided by carefully monitoring response to treatment and not decreasing treatment until good control has been established. Once again this can best be checked by regular peak flow recordings, particularly first thing in the morning or on waking at night (Fig. 2.4). Groups at particular risk are shown in the table below.

Asthmatics at particular risk

- Those with previous severe attacks, particularly if onset was sudden
- Those with a large diurnal variation of peak expiratory flow rate
- Asthmatics recently discharged from hospital
- In hospital, those recently discharged from intensive care
- Patients who require oral steroids
- Those with poor appreciation of changes in airway calibre

INHERITANCE

Both genetic and environmental factors are involved in the expression of asthma. The genetic factors are well illustrated in the Atlantic Island of Tristan de Cunha where the high prevalence of asthma can be traced back to three asthmatic females in the original settlers. Interestingly, asthma remains more common along females on the island, and two-thirds are intrinsic asthmatics with little atopy. The importance of environmental factors has been shown in a number of studies. For example, 3.2 per cent of Xhosa children living in Cape Town have asthma compared with 0.1 of Xhosa children in the rural area of Transkei.[26]

Family studies have confirmed that relatives of asthmatic patients have an increased prevalence of asthma.[27] They are also more likely to have eczema, hay fever and asymptomatic bronchial lability. These features are more common among the relatives of extrinsic than of intrinsic asthmatics. It is thought that the atopic status (positive skin-prick tests, hay fever, eczema) is inherited independently of a susceptibility to asthma. Atopy acts to increase the likelihood that the susceptibility to asthma will be expressed when the two coincide. There is considerable debate about a finding that atopy may be linked to chromosome 11q.[28]

Airway hyperresponsiveness may also have a genetic basis so the combination of a predisposition to atopy and hyperresponsiveness will further increase the risk of asthma. A number of different genes may be linked to hyperresponsiveness and tendency to IgE production. Links have been found with chromosome 11q[28] and with chromosome 6 and other links are being found which provide growing evidence of the polygenic nature of asthma inheritance. Polymorphisms can also be found which may explain some differences in response to therapy.

It has been suggested that breast feeding may reduce the chances of development of asthma and other atopic diseases by decreasing the exposure to allergens during the first few months of life.[29] There are some studies which have not confirmed these findings but, with its other advantages, it seems sensible to encourage breast feeding, particularly where one or both parents are atopic or asthmatic.

The birth order may be important in determining risk of asthma. First or second born children appear to be more likely to develop asthma. This may be because later children are more likely to have their immune system stimulated by exposure to common viral infections from their siblings during the first months of life.

THE RELATIONSHIP WITH CHRONIC AIRFLOW OBSTRUCTION

Certain asthmatic patients who show improvement with bronchodilators gradually lose this reversibility as they grow older. This is most likely to occur with poorly controlled severe asthma and is a function of the duration of the disease.[30] Such patients may also become chronic sputum producers and fit into the generally accepted definition of chronic bronchitis:

> Production of purulent sputum for at least three months of two consecutive years.

However, this progression to chronic airflow obstruction with little or no reversibility with beta$_2$ agonists is uncommon among nonsmoking asthmatics. These patients often still retain the ability to reverse with vigorous treatment, such as a course of oral corticosteroids. This exposure to two weeks of 40 mg of prednisolone per day, or the equivalent, should be regarded as essential before patients are consigned to the irreversible obstruction category.

Simple chronic bronchitis – cough and sputum without obstruction – seems to be little more than a harmless marker of tobacco smoking. By themselves cough and spit are not associated with a poor prognosis. Only those who have accompanying airflow obstruction run the progressively downhill course to respiratory failure. Some of the patients presenting in this way will have valuable reversibility. Even after ruling out improvement with an inhaled bronchodilator, 10 per cent will respond well to treatment such as corticosteroids and some of these may regain normal lung function.

Whether we choose to call these patients asthmatics or wheezy bronchitics is not really relevant. The important message is that we have to give them a chance to show their ability to improve by giving them the right treatment with bronchodilators and steroids.

SMOKING

Cigarette smoking provokes bronchoconstriction, particularly in asthmatics. Despite this, a significant number of asthmatics continue to smoke, probably about 15–20 per cent, over half the national average for England and Wales. They should be strongly discouraged from doing so because, apart from the other harmful effects of cigarette smoking, their asthma is likely to be easier to control without the persistent inhalation of irritating cigarette smoke.[31] There has also been the suggestion that it is asthmatic smokers, or those with reactive airways, who are most likely to be among the 20 to 25 per cent of smokers who go on to develop chronic airflow obstruction.[32] More detailed advice on helping patients to give up the habit is included in Chapter 11.

PRACTICAL POINTS

- Certain features about the onset of asthma in childhood can be used to predict whether a child will 'grow out of it'. The following are all associated with a poorer prognosis:
  – Severity at onset
  – Persistent symptoms
  – Frequent severe symptoms
  – Onset below three years
  – Associated atopic disease
  Nevertheless asthma generally improves through adolescence, especially in boys.
- Adult asthma tends to be more persistent, with less variability and less likelihood of remission.
- Asthma is associated with a great number of lost days from school and work. Adequate treatment and education of patients in adjustments of treatment should avoid such problems in the majority of patients.
- Mortality studies in asthma show that the great majority of deaths are related to inadequate treatment, because the true severity of the attack has not been appreciated by the patient or the physician.
- Both genetic and environmental factors are involved in the expression of asthma.
- Approximately a fifth to a quarter of asthmatics smoke cigarettes. They should be vigorously encouraged to give up the habit, both to promote the efficacy of treatment and to help prevent them developing chronic airflow obstruction.

3
Precipitating factors in asthma

BACKGROUND

Some acute exacerbations of asthma have obvious precipitating factors which patients recognize for themselves. This is most common with exposure to animals or seasonal allergens such as grass pollens. In more chronic persistent cases specific precipitating factors are less obvious. Precipitating factors such as grass pollen are so widespread in the environment that avoiding contact with them is not practical. In other cases, such as particular animal sensitivities, simple avoidance may prevent acute exacerbations.

It is important to identify such cases, as avoidance of the provoking factors is preferable to suppression of the effects by drug treatment. Usually these sensitivities can be identified through a careful clinical history, but skin tests and measurement of specific IgE can provide supportive evidence (see Chapter 8).

In practice, it is unusual to find that a single provoking agent is involved in a patient's asthma. Usually there are several factors which can stimulate the reactive airways. Specific allergens and general irritants can interact. The exposure to agents to which the subject is sensitive can induce hyperreactivity to nonspecific irritants and dusts. Avoiding the specific agent can lead to a gradual reduction in the reactivity of the airways and produce general improvement.

This chapter discusses the common provoking factors in asthma and how they can best be dealt with. Desensitization is considered further in Chapter 8.

The important inhaled allergens vary in different areas of the world and physicians should be aware of the major local allergens and their particular seasons (see Fig. 3.1).

INFECTION

Respiratory infections are the commonest factors claimed as precipitating acute attacks of asthma. The majority of these infections are of viral origin[33] and, therefore, antibiotics are inappropriate in their treatment. Rhinoviruses are the most common followed by parainfluenza and adenoviruses. Increased reactivity of the airways can be demonstrated for up to six weeks after viral infections in normal subjects and the same thing occurs in asthmatic patients.

Bacterial infections can precipitate attacks but not commonly enough to recommend antibiotics as a routine part of the treatment of acute asthma. The two bacteria most likely

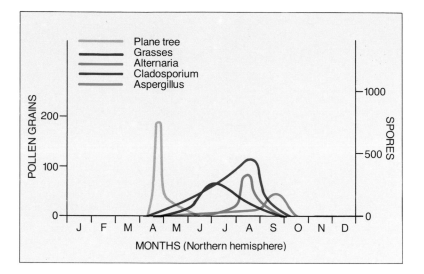

Figure 3.1 Seasonal distribution of pollens and mould spores in London.

to be involved are *Streptococcus pneumoniae* and *Haemophilus influenzae*, both of which are likely to respond to ampicillin, amoxycillin, tetracycline or co-trimoxazole.

It is best to reserve such antibiotics for acute exacerbations with reasonable evidence of infection. Green sputum may not be reliable as it may be packed with eosinophils rather than neutrophils. Airway responses to allergens can mimic infections with upper airway and systemic symptoms, coloured sputum and even fever. The diagnosis usually relies upon a convincing history with or without evidence of pulmonary shadowing on the chest X-ray. There is no place for long-term prophylactic antibiotic treatment in asthma.

Viral infections in infancy may be a trigger for asthma in the future. Over 50 per cent of children developing respiratory syncytial virus infections in infancy go on to have further episodes of wheezing during childhood.

HOUSE DUST MITES

House dust mites (Fig. 3.2) are very widely distributed throughout the Western world. *Dermatophagoides pteronyssinus* is mainly found in household dust, soft furnishings, bedding and soft toys. House dust mites provide the most common positive skin test in Britain, being positive in 80 per cent of children with severe asthma. The major allergen (Der P1) is found in the mites' faecal pellets. The mites thrive best in warm, damp conditions, so in dry cold climates, at altitudes above 1,500 metres and in desert environments they are much less common. Energy-saving house insulation tends to increase indoor humidity and leads to higher house dust mite concentrations.

It has been suggested that early exposure to increased mite numbers in homes may be partly responsible for the rise in the prevalence of asthma. Some studies have found that

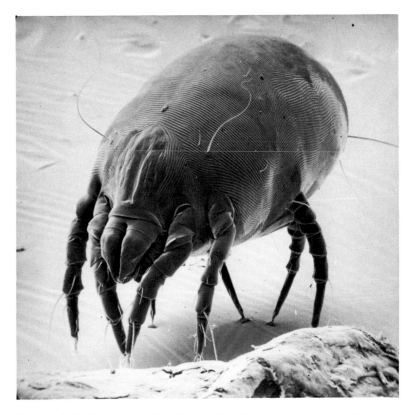

Figure 3.2 The house dust mite, *Dermatophagoides pteronyssinus*, provides a positive skin test in 80 per cent of children with severe asthma.

mite allergic subjects are more likely to be born in the later months of the year when mite levels are higher. Work from Australia suggests that while the underlying rate of atopy has not increased, mite numbers have gone up and the effect of this is shown by a rise in the number of subjects with symptoms of asthma.[34]

Adapting the home

The mites are so widespread that total eradication from the home is not possible. Patients are often advised to attack the mites vigorously in the asthmatic's bedroom. This includes the use of synthetic rather than feather pillows and duvets, enclosing mattresses, regular changing of bed-linen and vacuum cleaning of mattresses, bed-linen, curtains and so on. There is little point in pursuing these elaborate measures and then allowing the child to go to bed with an old dusty teddy bear! It is certainly worth trying to keep dust levels as low as possible in the bedroom.

Gore-tex mattress covers are expensive but are impervious to mites and their faecal particles, and these mattresses can be shown to reduce the allergen load. Vacuum cleaners can also be fitted with filters which remove the mite products rather than redistributing them around the room. Other measures such as the application of liquid nitrogen to mattresses can markedly reduce mite numbers for months. Anti-mite agents (acaricides) may also help. In mite-allergic subjects with troublesome asthma it is worth trying such measures, and if they improve asthma control then they are worth continuing.

There is no doubt that a very substantial reduction in the house dust mite is beneficial in some subjects. For instance, admission to hospital rooms that can be washed down regularly produces improvement.[35] Drastic measures are often not practical in the home environment.

Hyposensitization

Trials of hyposensitization have given conflicting results but there may be some benefit in certain children who have symptoms closely related to house dust mite exposure.[36,37] It is quite possible that further developments of vaccines may improve the results of hyposensitization. However, in the majority of children with symptoms related to one major factor such as house dust mites, control is easily obtained with simple pharmacological therapy (see Chapter 8). Where this is not possible a number of provocative factors are usually involved and hyposensitization to only one of them is not useful.

POLLENS

Grass pollens

These are the most important pollens in relation to hay fever and asthma in Europe and Australia. They are most abundant between late spring and midsummer. Some asthmatics have strictly seasonal wheezing but this is rarely very troublesome. It is more common to see perennial symptoms with other triggering factors and then exacerbations during the pollen season. Many grasses are antigenically similar: those most often causing problems are Bermuda, cocksfoot, couch, fescue, rye, timothy and sweet vernal (Figs 3.3–3.8).

Grass pollen is such an abundant substance that avoidance is possible only by the use of some sort of mask to filter out the pollen grains (size 15–60 µm). This is a totally impractical approach for most hay fever sufferers. The alternatives are pharmacological treatment (see Chapter 9) or hyposensitization (see Chapter 8).

Hyposensitization Although some trials show no benefit and there is a large placebo effect, hyposensitization probably has some effect in allergic rhinitis.[36] In pollen-sensitive asthma the benefit is less certain. The hyposensitization course needs to be given before the pollen season and there is some evidence of increasing benefits when courses are repeated over three or four years.

Occasionally severe reactions occur to hyposensitization injections, and, rarely fatalities result. These are almost always related to inappropriate dosage or route of injection. This treatment should be restricted to patients who have distinctly pollen-related asthma which is not easily controlled by other means. Patients must be observed carefully for at least one hour after each injection; and antihistamines, hydrocortisones and adrenaline, as well as resuscitation facilities, should be immediately available to deal with any reactions (see also Chapter 8).

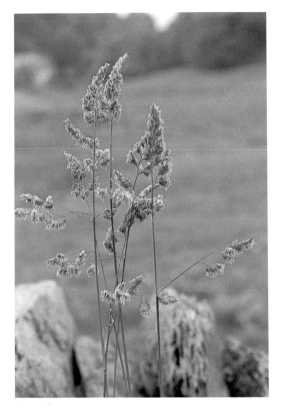

Figure 3.3 Cocksfoot grass.

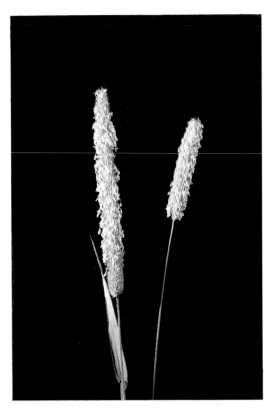

Figure 3.4 Timothy grass.

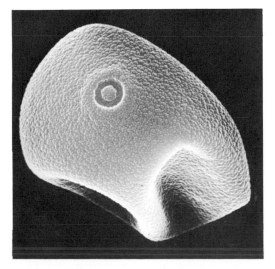

Figure 3.5 A scanning electron micrograph of a cocksfoot grass pollen grain (Mag: x 5,500).

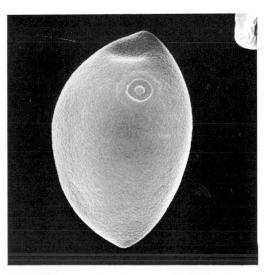

Figure 3.6 A scanning electron micrograph of a timothy grass pollen grain (Mag: x 3,800).

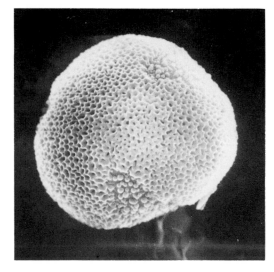

Figure 3.7 A scanning electron micrograph of a plane tree pollen grain (Mag: x 50,000).

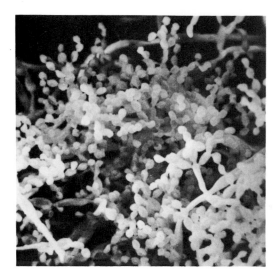

Figure 3.8 A scanning electron micrograph of a spore of Cladosporium (Mag: x 600).

Other pollens and spores

Seasonal symptoms which do not fit into the grass pollen season of late spring to midsummer may be produced by other pollens or spores, such as tree pollens or mould spores. As with grass pollen the symptoms produced are more commonly rhinitis and conjunctivitis than asthma.

When symptoms occur in early spring then tree pollen may be responsible, especially silver birch or plane pollen. Problems occurring predominantly in late summer may be produced by mould spores, most commonly *Alternaria tenuis*. *Alternaria* often grows on grain. Cladosporium grows on rotting vegetation and is the commonest mould spore, with a longer season than *Alternaria*, but is less often associated with symptoms. Skin tests provide useful confirmation of sensitivities to these seasonal allergens (see Chapter 8).

ANIMALS

Most animals that are kept as household pets are capable of causing problems with asthma. Doctors are often asked whether resident family pets should be removed or if new pets may be acquired when one of the children has asthma.

The question of new pets is easier. It is unwise for parents of asthmatic children to acquire a cat, dog, horse, rodent or bird. Sensitivity and positive skin tests can soon develop with close animal contact. A negative skin test or RAST (radioallergosorbent test) for IgE before exposure or soon after the pet arrives are no guarantee that problems will not occur in the future.

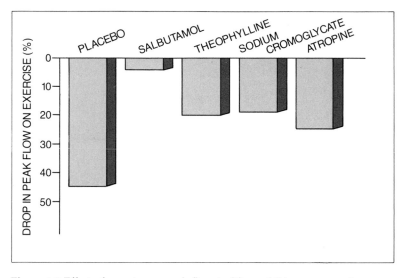

Figure 3.9 Effect of exercise on peak flow in fifteen children expressed as percentage change from pre-exercise values. Salbutamol, theophylline and atropine all produced an initial bronchodilatation.

If pets are already in the home, the situation is less clear cut. They are unlikely to be the only agent provoking asthma, so the effect of removal is difficult to predict. Getting rid of a loved family pet can provoke emotional problems in children which themselves make the asthma worse. There must, therefore, be good reasons for removing an established pet. These come from a demonstration of the effects of exposure to the pet. The decision to remove the pet is not really influenced by a positive skin test although it would be surprising to encounter pet-induced problems in the presence of a negative skin test.

A history of wheezing in relation to exposure should lead to a trial separation of animal and asthmatic. This usually has to be done by temporary removal of the asthmatic rather than the animal, since the allergen will stay around the house for some time after the animal has gone. Trials of exposure and removal are monitored by peak flow records and changes in the frequency of bronchodilator treatment.

Cats are the most frequent source of trouble, with allergens in urine, saliva, hair and dander. The allergens seem to be the same in most cats except perhaps Siamese. Dogs show greater differences between species. Horses, birds and all of the small rodents can also produce adverse effects.

EXERCISE

Formal exercise tests produce a diagnostic drop in peak flow or FEV$_1$ in most asthmatic patients. A smaller number of patients complain of troublesome wheezing after exertion and it is unusual for this to be the sole asthmatic stimulus. Fortunately exercise-induced asthma can usually be avoided easily by the use of a beta$_2$ agonist or sodium cromoglycate just before exercise (Fig. 3.9). Nedocromil sodium has a similar blocking effect.

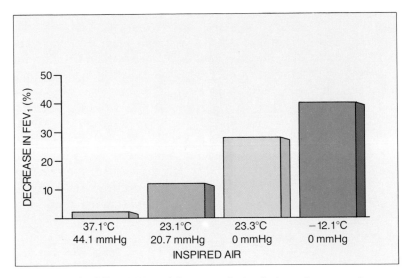

Figure 3.10 The fall in FEV$_1$ with hyperventilation is dependent upon the temperature of the inspired air. Similar relationships are seen with exercise-induced bronchoconstriction.

Anticholinergic drugs and theophylline are rather less successful in the control of exercise-induced asthma. Single doses of inhaled corticosteroids do not prevent wheezing but regular treatment appears to be effective.

Calcium antagonists, frusemide and antihistamines have some effect in studies of exercise-induced asthma but they do not have a practical role.

The mechanisms of exercise-induced asthma

A great deal has been learned about these over the last few years. Recent work has explained some earlier clinical observations of the types of exercise most likely to induce asthma.[38] A large part of the stimulus in exercise-induced asthma comes from cooling and drying of the airway epithelium by the inspired air (Fig. 3.10).[14] Because of the increase in ventilation the air is no longer fully warmed and saturated as it is at rest. Exercise-induced asthma can be mimicked by breathing the same quantity of cold, dry air without the physical exertion. Increase in osmolality of the mucosa and lining fluid appears to be the most important factor.

The way in which cooling and drying of the mucosa produces bronchoconstriction is still unclear. Rises in histamine and neutrophil chemotactic factor suggest that there is nonimmunological degranulation of mast cells.

Exercise-induced asthma can be avoided by breathing warm, moist air during exertion. This may explain the observation that swimming, particularly in heated indoor pools, is less of a stimulus to asthma than running. Schoolchildren find that outdoor exercises on a cold winter morning are the most potent stimulus to their asthma.

Which sports are least problematic?

Although exercise and training are not likely to be of much direct benefit in control of asthma, fitness is as desirable for asthmatics as it is for the rest of us. Asthmatics looking for a sport to take up might be advised to choose swimming as the least potent stimulus. Several centres have started up swimming groups to encourage exercise and fitness in asthmatic children. On rare occasions, the situation with swimming is complicated by sensitivity to chlorine which can induce asthma. Sports which involve short bursts of exercise, such as cricket, produce fewer symptoms than sustained activity, as in middle- and long-distance running. However, simple medication with an inhaled beta$_2$ agonist before exertion will allow asthmatics to take part in most sports if their control is otherwise good. Schoolchildren should be encouraged to take part in sports with this pretreatment. They can then stay fit and lead normal school lives rather than being unduly protected because of their asthma.

With the growing problems of drug administration in athletics and other sports, asthmatics must be aware of any restrictions. In some situations, any drugs prescribed by a doctor are allowed. The International Olympic Committee allows salbutamol and terbutaline, cromoglycate, nedocromil sodium and inhaled corticosteroids, but competitors should inform the authorities about the need for such drugs.

SMOKING

The hyperreactivity of asthmatic airways makes them likely to constrict in response to nonspecific stimuli such as dusts. Cigarette smoke is a potent stimulus for many asthmatic patients, and yet around 20 per cent of asthmatics continue to smoke. As we have said, this should be strongly discouraged. Not only does it lead to difficulties in asthmatic control but asthmatics may well be particularly likely to go on to get chronic airflow obstruction. Apart from the personal air pollution of asthmatic cigarette smokers, some patients find problems in smoky atmospheres. They are victims of passive smoking.[39]

There is evidence that maternal smoking during pregnancy and during infant life increases the chance of asthmatic problems in the children.[40]

More general air pollution can also be troublesome. Asthmatics are sensitive to much lower concentrations of pollutants, such as sulphur dioxide, than normal individuals.

POLLUTION

Exercise at times of high pollution levels is especially likely to give problems. Many areas produce regular pollution reports and asthmatic symptoms increase with higher levels of oxides of nitrogen and particulates. Patients with asthma or other lung problems may be advised to avoid exercise outdoors when levels are high.

Several studies have suggested that asthma symptoms increase in association with pollution levels. Asthma symptoms and attendances at Accident and Emergency Departments have been linked to high levels of respirable particulates, ozone, SO_2 and NO_2.

Climatic changes such as atmospheric pressure drops at the time of thunderstorms can bring pollen grains and other allergens down from higher in the atmosphere and provoke marked increases in exacerbations of asthma.

Asthmatic patients are well advised to avoid dusty atmospheres. It is best not to choose an occupation, such as building work, where dust levels are high. Such nonspecific irritation at work can maintain airway hyperreactivity and interfere with control.

DRUGS

Many drugs have been associated with precipitation of asthma. The two groups most commonly recognized are beta blockers and the nonsteroidal anti-inflammatory drugs (NSAIDs).

Drugs inducing asthma

- Beta blockers
- NSAIDs
- Iodine-based contrast media
- Dextrans
- Dyes and preservatives used in drug formulation
- Antibiotics
  - Nitrofurantoin
  - Penicillin
  - Tetracycline
  - Streptomycin
  - Erythromycin
  - Griseofulvin
- Sulphasalazine
- Carbamazepine
- Pituitary snuff
- Mineral oil

Beta blockers

These often produce adverse effects when given to asthmatics. Treatment with beta blockers can also bring to light previously undiagnosed asthma. Fatal bronchoconstriction has been produced by a single dose of beta blockers. Even administration as timolol eye drops in glaucoma has given trouble. Beta blockers such as metoprolol and atenolol are more cardioselective and slightly less likely to cause trouble in asthmatics. Nevertheless, they certainly cannot be regarded as safe for them. The cardioselective drugs have the advantage that any bronchoconstriction can normally be reversed by beta$_2$ agonists, although very much larger doses than usual are likely to be necessary.[43]

It is best to avoid all beta blockers in asthmatics. Fortunately, calcium channel blockers are an alternative treatment for hypertension and angina. They do not cause bronchoconstriction and may even act to prevent exercise-induced asthma.[44,45]

NSAIDs

Around 2 per cent of adult asthmatics have problems with aspirin and other NSAIDs. On formal testing, bronchoconstriction is much more common after aspirin.[46]

The mechanism seems to be related to the action of the drugs in blocking prostaglandin production. Prostaglandins are produced by cyclo-oxygenation of arachidonic acid, derived from phospholipids in cell membranes. Blockade of this pathway increases the activity of the lipoxygenase pathway, by which arachidonic acid is metabolized to leukotrienes which produce bronchoconstriction. The importance of the aspirin reaction lies in identifying it and then making sure that the patient avoids the other drugs in the group, such as indomethacin, naproxen, diclofenac, and so on. It is possible to achieve desensitization to aspirin by gradually increasing oral doses of aspirin under careful supervision.

Other types of drugs and treatments

Drugs such as penicillin, which sometimes cause anaphylactic reactions, can produce asthma as part of these reactions. Asthma has been recorded with many other drugs which can be seen in the table on page 36.

Angiotensin-converting enzyme inhibitors such as captopril and enalapril produce a persistent dry cough in around 5% of patients. This may be related to their prevention of breakdown of kinins such as bradykinin in the airway epithelium. However, development or worsening of asthma is unusual.[47]

Bronchoconstriction produced by asthma treatment

1. **Nonspecific irritant effect**
   - Dry powder delivery system

2. **Effect of deep inspiration**

3. **Specific sensitivity to drug**
   - Bromide moeity in ipratropium bromide
   - Theophylline
   - Ethylenediamine in aminophylline
   - Hydrocortisone

4. **Propellants, preservatives**
   - Contaminants from valve in metered dose inhalers
   - Preservatives in nebulizer solutions

5. **Nebulization of hypotonic solutions**

Many of the preparations used in the treatment of asthma can produce inappropriate bronchoconstriction on occasions (see table above). This can occur as a nonspecific reaction to the dry powder of sodium cromoglycate, steroids or bronchodilators. Ipratropium bromide can produce reproducible reactions said to be caused by a sensitivity to the bromide constituent.[48] Reactions to beta$_2$ agonists are much less common; they are most often related to contaminants from the valve apparatus of the metered dose inhaler. Aminophylline can produce sensitivity reactions either to theophylline itself or to the ethylenediamine component. Even intravenous hydrocortisone has induced generalized reactions involving airway obstruction. Bronchoconstrictor responses to nebulizers have been related to preservatives in the solutions and to the hypotonicity. Ipratropium bromide is now produced as an isotonic, preservative-free nebulizer solution. Other drugs delivered by nebulizer (e.g. pentamidine for treatment or prophylaxis of pneumocystis pneumonia) may also provoke airway narrowing.

Physical forms of treatment such as haemodialysis can also, rarely, be associated with asthmatic exacerbations.

FOODS

'Food allergy' has generated a great deal of interest from the press and television. Many dubious claims have been made about the importance of allergic reactions to food. 'Food intolerance' is a better term than 'food allergy' as it makes no assumptions about the mechanisms involved.[49] Asthmatic reactions to food are easier to prove or disprove than some more general responses such as changes in mood or arthralgia.

Where responses to food have been assessed in an objective and controlled manner, the results usually fail to substantiate many of the original claims of food sensitivity. Nevertheless some asthmatics do have consistent and sometimes severe reactions to foods.[49] Many foods have been incriminated in this way, but reactions are most common in children, occur within the first hour of ingestion and are usually associated with other allergic features such as urticaria, rhinitis and increased bowel activity. Sulphur dioxide in some commercially produced soft drinks such as orange squash and fizzy drinks can produce bronchoconstriction by an irritant effect.

Milk, nuts, alcoholic drinks and the yellow colouring agent, tartrazine, produce reactions most frequently. Tartrazine is widely used and is even found in some antihistamines which may be given as treatment for other signs of sensitivity. Nuts, including peanuts (which are legumes rather than true nuts) can provoke dramatic asthma which may be fatal. Sensitive patients need to be very careful to avoid even small quantities used in cooking.

Because most food reactions occur early rather than late, the patient very often has recognized the food responsible. Skin tests are of little use in confirmation. Occasionally dairy or cereal products produce later reactions, sometimes obvious only when the product has been excluded from the diet for a week or two. It is always worth carefully asking the patient about any suspicions he may have regarding diet, but elaborate exclusion diets rarely produce results and are not recommended.

Foods most commonly involved in asthmatic reactions

- Milk
- Eggs
- Nuts
- Alcoholic drinks
- Sulphur dioxide
- Tartrazine

OCCUPATION

There has been increasing recognition of occupational asthma over the last few years.[50] Occupational factors are important in about 5 per cent of cases of asthma beginning in adults. In Britain occupational asthma has been legally recognized as a compensatable industrial disease since 1982. The substances listed in the table below are recognized for such compensation; the original list of seven was expanded in 1986. Other agents medically recognized as causes of occupational asthma are shown in the table on page 40, and are not yet included in the legislation. The number compensated under the legislation is relatively small and suggests underdiagnosis of occupational factors.

Workers at most risk

The mechanisms involved in occupational asthma are of great interest and may help in understanding the aetiology of other forms of asthma. In some cases a large proportion of exposed workers develop asthma. For example, more than half the workers exposed to complex platinum salts in some platinum refineries developed asthma. Other agents such as wood dust, enzymes or antibiotics produce occupational asthma in a much smaller proportion of exposed workers.

Workers who are atopic but with no history of asthma are at increased risk of developing occupational asthma in many industries. This is the case for workers exposed to enzyme detergents and to laboratory animals such as rats, but not for those exposed to isocyanates; and it raises the possibility that, fearing claims for compensation, some industries might screen job applicants to exclude from employment those with positive skin tests or a history of atopy.

Occupational asthma: substances legally recognized in Britain for industrial injury purposes

Substances	Workers likely to be at risk
• Platinum salts	• Platinum metal refiners
• Isocyanates	• Polyurethane foam makers; adhesive, rubber and print workers
• Epoxy resins	• Adhesive, paint and plastic workers
• Colophony (rosin) fumes	• Electronic solderers
• Proteolytic enzymes	• Biological detergent and chemical workers
• Laboratory animals and insects	• Laboratory workers and breeders
• Grain or flour dust	• Farmers, millers and bakers
• Wood dusts	• Carpenters, woodyard workers
• Drug manufacture (antibiotics, ispaghula, cimetidine, ipecacuanha)	• Pharmaceutical workers
• Castor bean dust	• Castor oil refining workers
• Azodicarbonamide	• Plastic blowing

Other medically recognized causes of occupational asthma

- Pollens
- Green coffee beans
- Tobacco and tea
- Micro-organisms and humidifiers
- Mushrooms
- Silk
- Dyes

- Gum acacia
- Cotton
- Metal (chromates, cobalt, nickel, vanadium)
- PVC
- Formaldehyde
- Ethylenediamine
- Hairdressing solutions

Testing for occupational asthma

Occupational asthma should be considered in all adults whether or not there is an obvious relationship between wheezing and work. The first step in investigation of a possible relationship is to obtain a peak flow record during time at and away from work.

A relationship may be immediately obvious when an instant reaction occurs on exposure (Fig. 3.11). Such reactions may be so obvious that further challenge testing with the material in the laboratory will not be necessary unless it is a question of sorting out which agent at work is involved. In other cases reactions may be delayed, appearing later in the day at work or in the evening or at night after work. These reactions become more obvious when peak flow records over a weekend at home show improvement.

Sometimes a more difficult pattern occurs in which peak flows are consistently low and fail to improve over weekend breaks. These patients may need a week or two away from exposure before there is evidence of improvement. In these cases a definite relationship is more difficult to establish (Fig. 3.12).

Where there is doubt about the existence of occupational asthma or about which agent is involved, then challenge testing in the laboratory may be necessary (Fig. 3.13). This should be done only under close supervision in an experienced laboratory. An attempt should be made to mimic work exposure as closely as possible and patients must be observed over the time during which any late reaction might occur (usually for 24 hours).

Latent reactions

Many patients may deny that occupational factors can be involved, because they have been doing the same job for many years, but this is no protection. With colophony, a substance derived from pine resin and used as a soldering flux, ten years of exposure may elapse before a reaction is experienced, the median lag period being more than four years. These lag periods tend to be shorter in patients who already have a history of asthma.

Exposure at work can induce nonspecific hyperreactivity which produced problems in general asthma control. Asthma does not necessarily disappear on removal from exposure, particularly if the occupational contact has been prolonged. There may be persistent airflow obstruction and reactions to other provoking stimuli such as exercise and infections are common.

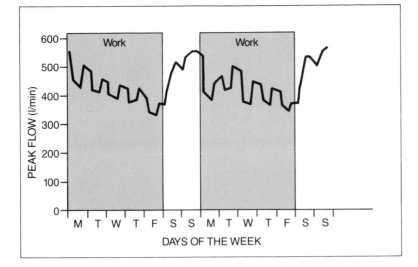

Figure 3.11 Immediate occupational reactions occur on each day at work but often show a progressive deterioration during the working week.

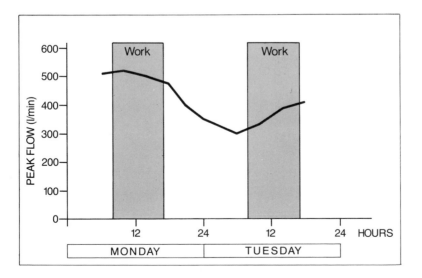

Figure 3.12 Late asthmatic reactions such as the responses shown may be more difficult to relate to occupation since the greatest airway narrowing occurs away from the workplace.

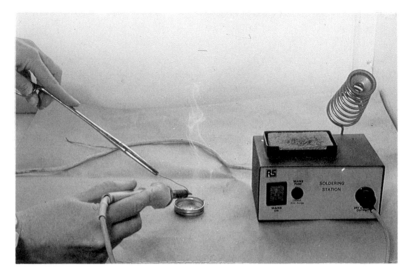

Figure 3.13 Challenge tests in the laboratory. The patient is using a multicore solder which contains colophony. Measurements of airflow are made for at least six hours after exposure to detect early and late responses.

Compensation

In Britain, for the purposes of compensation, the Industrial Injuries Advisory Council defines occupational asthma as 'asthma which develops after a variable period of symptomless exposure to a sensitizing agent at work'. Only specific sensitizing agents are the subject of compensation (those listed in the table on page 39). Nonspecific irritation by dust, smoke or sulphur dioxide would not be considered. Assessment for compensation is by way of the Medical Boarding Centre and further information can be found in the document produced by the Industrial Advisory Council or from local DSS offices.[51]

PSYCHOLOGICAL FACTORS

Emotional factors are usually considered to be important in asthma. In acute severe asthma the sensation of breathlessness is very frightening and often provokes marked anxiety. Generally, psychological factors are most likely to be important when control of asthma is poor. This is certainly the case in children, where emotional problems between parents and children are increased only in the severe group. If these problems can be sorted out, asthma control often improves.

The two components, severe asthma and psychological factors, are likely to be closely interrelated. While persistent disease may increase emotional problems, personality difficulties may lead to poor compliance with treatment and poorer control. Therefore, it may be difficult to disentangle the two. There is, though, no evidence that emotional or psychological factors predispose to the development of asthma, nor that psychological

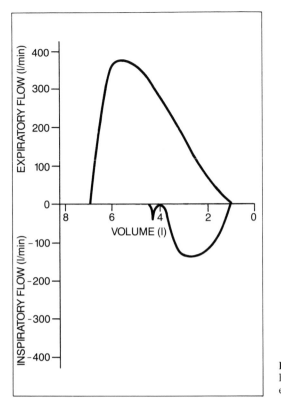

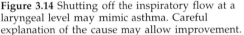

Figure 3.14 Shutting off the inspiratory flow at a laryngeal level may mimic asthma. Careful explanation of the cause may allow improvement.

factors can be the sole cause of asthma. Nevertheless, any significant psychiatric abnormalities should be treated at the same time as the asthma.

Placebo effect

Appropriate suggestion can influence either the bronchodilator or bronchoconstrictor effect during laboratory experiments and clinical trials.[52] A placebo can be made to produce either effect with suitable encouragement. These effects of suggestion probably explain therapeutic successes with acupuncture and hypnosis (see Chapter 10).

Upper airway obstruction masquerading as asthma

Some patients who have mild or no asthma, can have wheezing from upper airway obstruction at a laryngeal level (Fig. 3.14).[53] This may be difficult to differentiate from an acute attack of asthma. The wheezing is mainly inspiratory and the site of obstruction can usually be best seen in a flow volume loop. Between attacks these patients usually have normal bronchial reactivity. The attacks may come at times of anxiety and such patients often have emotional or psychiatric problems. Exploration of the problem and psychiatric support may be helpful but management is often difficult.

PREGNANCY AND MENSTRUATION

Pregnancy has a variable effect upon asthmatic control. During pregnancy about a third of patients show significant improvement, while a similar proportion experience a significant deterioration.[54] There are naturally worries about drug treatment in pregnancy. Corticosteroids increase congenital defects such as cleft palate in animals. However, poorly controlled asthma and accompanying hypoxia are more of a threat to pregnancy, so such treatments should not be withheld if they are indicated. Inhaled beta$_2$ agonists, sodium cromoglycate and ipratropium bromide are regularly used in normal doses in pregnancy and are not thought to add any significant risk.

Asthma may worsen in time with menstruation in about one-third of women, but the deterioration is not usually very severe (see Chapter 11).

GASTRO-OESOPHAGEAL REFLUX

Occasionally gastro-oesophageal reflux is an important trigger factor in asthma. This is particularly likely to be a problem at night. Bronchoconstriction may be produced by spillage of acid into the larynx or upper airways. There is some evidence also of a reflex bronchoconstrictor response to acid in the lower oesophagus.[55]

When there is evidence of gastro-oesophageal reflux in asthmatic patients it should be treated appropriately. Both medical and surgical treatment can lead to improvement in asthmatic control in such individuals.

THYROID DISEASE

There are a number of causes of shortness of breath in thyrotoxicosis. One of these is the worsening or development of asthma. The mechanism is unclear. The commonest situation is the worsening of established asthma with the development of hyperthyroidism. Control then returns with treatment of the thyroid disease. Less common is improvement of asthma with the development of hypothyroidism. This, of course, has no place in treatment. Thyroxine replacement should be done carefully while the asthma is appropriately treated.

ALLERGIC BRONCHOPULMONARY ASPERGILLOSIS (ABPA)

ABPA, caused by sensitivity to the fungus *Aspergillus fumigatus*, is more a complication rather than a provocative factor of asthma. However, it is associated with acute exacerbations of asthma and therefore should be borne in mind as a possible precipitating factor. Being a sensitivity reaction, we cover the diagnosis, natural history and treatment of ABPA in Chapter 8, which deals with the immunological aspects of asthma.

PRACTICAL POINTS

- A few individuals have their asthmatic attacks precipitated by one specific agent. More commonly the reactive airways of an asthmatic are stimulated by many trigger factors.
- It is worth trying to identify important precipitating factors by a careful history. Any further investigations will follow on from suspicious features in the story. The first move is usually to confirm an association by the use of peak flow records at home or at work.
- In most cases the management consists of avoidance of the trigger factor or, when this is not possible, suppression of the symptoms by drug treatment. Specific desensitization is rarely appropriate because of the poor success rate and the potential dangers.
- Asthma developing in relation to occupation is the subject of compensation in many countries.
- Precipitating factors include:
  - Infection
  - House dust mites
  - Pollens
  - Animals
  - Exercise
  - Smoking
  - Dust and pollution
  - Drugs
  - Foods
  - Occupation
  - Psychological factors
  - Pregnancy and menstruation
  - Gastro-oesophageal reflux
  - Thyroid disease
  - Allergic bronchopulmonary aspergillosis (ABPA)

4
Management of acute asthma

BACKGROUND

As asthma is by nature a paroxysmal condition, acute attacks are its hallmark. The management of an attack of asthma depends to a large extent upon the severity of the attack and its response to treatment. Most acute episodes respond rapidly to an increase in treatment but some do not; and if the attack becomes persistent and intractable it is sometimes known as status asthmaticus or more commonly as acute severe asthma.

It is not known whether there is a different pathophysiological mechanism underlying those episodes of acute asthma which fail to respond to a conventional increase in therapy. Many speculate that when this occurs and status asthmaticus is diagnosed, mucosal oedema and mucus plugging play a more important role than bronchoconstriction, and hence the attack is more difficult to eradicate, being more resistant to bronchodilator therapy.

Treatment of an acute attack has two main goals:

1. To hasten recovery
2. To prevent the patient's asthma from spiralling down to a dangerous level when death may arise.

Prompt and effective treatment of asthmatic attacks may therefore help avert asthma deaths and this is discussed in detail below.

A severe attack of asthma should be regarded as a failure of control and previous treatment should be examined and changed to prevent a recurrence.

ASSESSMENT OF THE ATTACK

As treatment to a large extent depends on the severity of the attack it is important to be clear about the means of assessing the episode.

Clinical features

In general, clinical criteria are most helpful and provide the basis for such an assessment.

The patient will report an increase in symptoms with decreasing exercise tolerance and the appearance of dyspnoea at rest.

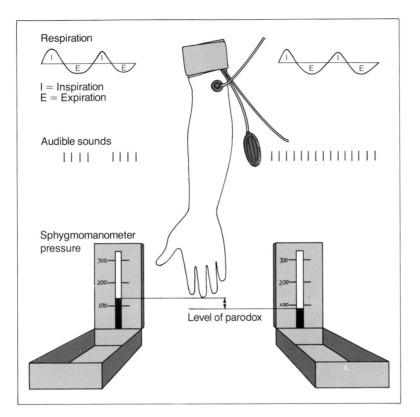

Respiration

I = Inspiration
E = Expiration

Audible sounds

Sphygmomanometer
pressure

Level of parodox

Figure 4.1 The measurement of the paradoxical pulse is a guide to the progress of an asthmatic attack. However, it may be absent even in severe asthma.

Sleep disturbance Of even greater importance is sleep disturbance by asthma. The patient will be woken earlier in the morning and then at intervals throughout the night as his condition deteriorates. In many asthmatics symptoms of sleep disturbance appear with fairly normal daytime exercise tolerance and represent the earliest sign of poor asthma control and require a review of treatment.

Increasing need for bronchodilator In addition to the symptoms becoming worse and more evidently diurnal, most patients also notice an increased need for their bronchodilator treatment combined with its diminishing effectiveness. Thus the patient will find that the early morning bronchodilator lasts for shorter and shorter periods of time and therefore more bronchodilator is being consumed earlier in the day. The number of occasions for which a bronchodilator is required increases and this is an important sign of deteriorating asthma.

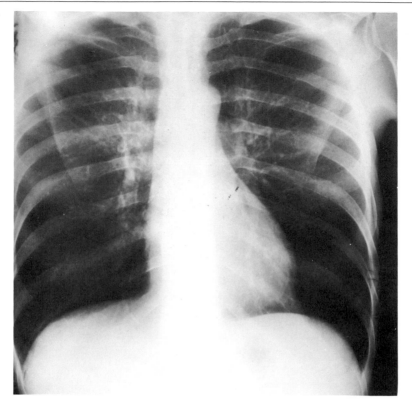

Figure 4.2 (a) Chest X-ray during an acute attack of asthma showing overinflation of the lungs.

Pathological features

Lung function In addition to these clinical features, the lung function of the patient will deteriorate. This is usually estimated by measuring peak expiratory flow (PEF) which can be recorded by the patient if he or she has a peak flow meter or by the practitioner when visiting the patient. The mean daily PEF will fall and often this is mainly the result of a marked fall in the early morning peak flow. If peak flow is measured on a number of occasions over the twenty-four hours a large amplitude change is observed with marked morning dips, but if the onset of the acute episode is very rapid this may be obscured by the rapid plummeting of the PEF.

Cardiovascular effects Acute asthma not only effects the respiratory system but most importantly the cardiovascular system as well. This is manifest by tachycardia, and when the attack is severe also by pulsus paradoxus.

It is very important not to ignore a pulse rate of over 110 beats per minute in an asthmatic patient complaining of an increase in symptoms. Although it is possible that the tachycardia may result from anxiety or administration of a nonselective broncho-dilator such as isoprenaline or aminophylline it is best to assume that the tachycardia reflects a severe attack of asthma.

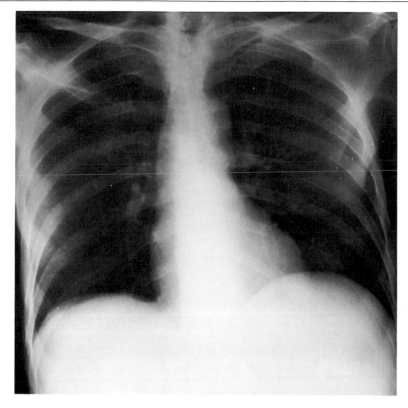

Figure 4.2 (b) The same patient as in the illustration opposite showing return of lung volumes to normal after recovery from the acute asthmatic attack.

If the pulse disappears when the patient breathes in, indicating a marked degree of pulsus paradoxus (Fig 4.1), this also suggests a severe attack of asthma, warranting intensive therapy. However, pulsus paradoxus may be absent even in very severe attacks of asthma. When present, the measurement, which is easily performed with a sphygmomanometer, provides a guide to progress and the response to treatment.[56]

Hospital tests

Other methods of assessment are usually best reserved for hospital care such as chest X-ray, blood gases and ECG. These are seldom necessary to identify a very severe attack of asthma as the clinical indices and measurement of PEF should suffice.

The chest X-ray is not usually helpful in the management of asthma. It usually just shows overinflation (Fig. 4.2). It is necessary to look for a pneumothorax if this is suspected (Fig. 4.3). Clinically this diagnosis may be difficult to exclude in acute exacerbations.

The ECG will show a tachycardia and may show signs of right ventricular strain or the development of a large P-wave, P pulmonale. These abnormalities will return to normal as the attack subsides (Fig. 4.4).

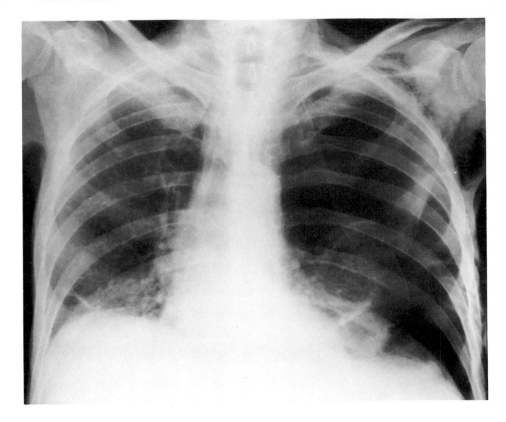

Figure 4.3 A pneumothorax is an unusual complication of acute asthma. However, when it does occur it may be difficult to detect on clinical examination of the chest.

Blood gases provide important information to help the management of severe asthma in hospital. The usual finding is of a low arterial PaO_2 and low $PaCO_2$. When the $PaCO_2$ is found to be high this should be a danger sign that the patient may be becoming tired and be likely to need assisted ventilation if immediate improvement cannot be achieved.

Warning signs of an acute attack

- Early warning signs
  - Sleep disturbance
  - Increase in symptoms
  - Decrease in exercise tolerance
  - Increasing need for bronchodilator treatment
  - Decreasing effectiveness of bronchodilator treatment
  - Fall in peak flow

- Signs of increasing severity
  - Dyspnoea at rest
  - Tachycardia
  - Pulsus paradoxus
  - Peak flow below 100 l/min
  - Abnormal blood gases

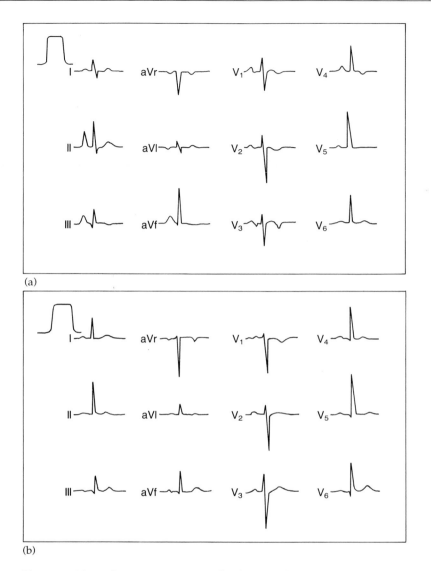

(a)

(b)

Figure 4.4 Many changes may occur in the electrocardiogram in acute asthma and then reverse on recovery. (a) In the acute state there is P pulmonale, a shift of the P-wave axis towards the right, a suggestion of right ventricular enlargement and anterior T-wave inversion. (b) These have returned to normal on the ECG taken after recovery.

PREVENTION OF A SEVERE ATTACK

Before considering treatment of an established attack of severe intractable asthma, it should be remembered that these attacks are best prevented and usually can be. Patients themselves can often recognize the warning signs, namely the onset of sleep disturbance and an increase in bronchodilator consumption. It is at this stage that a prompt increase in treatment may prevent a very severe attack of asthma from occurring. Much will depend upon the nature of the asthma and the background level of severity but usually all that is required at this stage is for treatment to be increased. If inhaled treatment is being used the dose can simply be doubled, but if only bronchodilators are being used it is essential to add anti-inflammatory medication.

Prednisolone therapy

If the attack supervenes very rapidly and is severe, a short course of prednisolone is required. It cannot be emphasized enough that this approach is safe and certainly much safer than a poorly controlled attack of asthma.

The usual mistake is either to delay the course of prednisolone or to give too small a dose for too short a period of time. In an otherwise fit and healthy adult, 45–60 mg per day can be tolerated quite satisfactorily and even in the oldest and most infirm patient, a minimum of 30 mg per day is probably necessary. This dose should last for at least one week; where there is any doubt, the high dose can be maintained for two weeks. Many patients are used to tailing the dose off although this has no benefit over a maintained steady dose and an abrupt stop. The course can last for up to three weeks without producing harmful systemic side-effects although some patients do notice early features of weight gain, and a diabetic with asthma may lose control of diabetes, which will then need to be managed separately.

Prompt and effective treatment at this stage will prevent most patients from developing status asthmaticus and this should be the practitioner's aim. Not only will this diminish the distress to the patient but it may also reduce or abolish risk of asthma death. On balance, asthma treatment is far safer than severe asthma.

TREATMENT OF AN ACUTE ATTACK

The treatment of an acute attack, like the prevention, will depend to a large extent upon its severity and the nature of the underlying asthma. It will also depend to a lesser extent on the long-term strategy for treating asthma, but we shall assume at this stage that the majority of patients are treated for most of the time with inhaled therapy. As discussed elsewhere, this provides effective treatment with the minimum dose and therefore the greatest safety margin for asthma management.

Bronchodilators

Most asthmatic patients will be receiving bronchodilators, usually by the inhaled route, but attacks can arise despite this treatment. In view of this it may seem paradoxical that most patients, particularly if admitted to hospital, will be treated first with inhaled bronchodilators via a nebulizer, usually with the same agents as taken at home, such as salbutamol. The reason why such an approach is often successful is not entirely clear but probably relates to three main factors:

1. The dose delivered is much higher than that taken by the patient via a conventional hand-held inhaler. For example, the usual starting dose of nebulized salbutamol is at least 2.5 mg, which is the equivalent of 25 puffs of salbutamol. Although a large proportion of this does not reach the

patient's lungs, approximately the same fraction hits the target as achieved by the pressurized aerosol and therefore the dose is very much higher.

2. Nebulizer therapy also helps as it is likely that many patients with severe asthma use their inhaler less effectively due to distress or panic. This may explain why supervised hand-held inhaler treatment by hospital staff or the use of a large volume spacer can achieve much better results than that obtained by the patients just before admission.

3. The inspiratory flow rate may be too low to take in the output of a metered dose inhaler adequately.

These considerations suggest that a higher dose of bronchodilator should be the first line of treatment, whether given by nebulizer or by more actuations of a hand-held device. The first approach to treating acute asthmatic attacks should therefore be to increase the inhaled dose.

Thus high-dose nebulized beta$_2$ agonist treatment represents the first step in the treatment of acute severe asthma. This approach is now incorporated into guidelines for asthma management (e.g. British Thoracic Society Guidelines, NIH International Consensus Report on the diagnosis and management of asthma).[57,58] If the response is suboptimal, nebulized ipratropium bromide can be added. This treatment in combination with a nebulized beta$_2$ agonist such as salbutamol can be more effective than treatment with the beta$_2$ agonist alone. In severe exacerbations bronchodilator nebulizations may need to be repeated every 15–30 minutes initially.

Aminophylline The use of intravenous aminophylline remains controversial. Undoubtedly it can provide effective bronchodilatation and may do so in patients who are not responding to inhaled beta$_2$ agonists. Unfortunately, aminophylline is a much less safe bronchodilator than others available today and it may cause death. This may occur if aminophylline is given too quickly or if too large a dose is given, particularly to a patient already on theophylline therapy. This problem is magnified if the patient is on long-term theophylline therapy delivered by a sustained-release preparation.[59]

If blood levels are not known, it is best either to avoid giving aminophylline or to err on the very cautious side. The initial loading dose should usually be 250 mg or 5 mg/kg up to a maximum of 350 mg. If theophyllines have been used by the patient before the attack, then the initial loading dose should be at least halved. The injection of the loading dose of aminophylline must be slow, taking at least fifteen minutes to complete.

If further doses are required it is again wise not to exceed 250 mg per injection and to limit these to a maximum of a further three or four over twenty-four hours. The need for further doses of aminophylline should be an indication that hospital admission is necessary. The aminophylline may then be continued by intravenous infusion initially at a rate of 0.5 mg/kg/h and monitored by drug levels (Fig. 4.5).

These doses are considerably smaller than are commonly employed but death may arise through theophylline toxicity, particularly in older patients. As safer alternative treatment is available, aminophylline treatment is best reserved for patients not previously taking xanthines, or for hospital when aminophylline blood level monitoring can be performed.

Associated renal or hepatic disease considerably increases the risks of toxicity. The most frequent side-effects of theophyllines are nausea and vomiting, but occasionally neurological or cardiovascular problems may occur with no such warning.

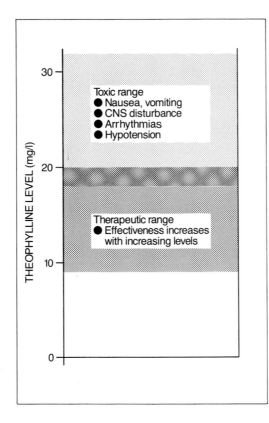

THEOPHYLLINE LEVEL (mg/l)

30 —

Toxic range
● Nausea, vomiting
● CNS disturbance
● Arrhythmias
● Hypotension

20 —

Therapeutic range
● Effectiveness increases
  with increasing levels

10 —

0 —

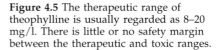

Figure 4.5 The therapeutic range of theophylline is usually regarded as 8–20 mg/l. There is little or no safety margin between the therapeutic and toxic ranges.

If the patient qualifies for aminophylline then normally they will also require a course of corticosteroids.

Corticosteroids

In a mild exacerbation, nebulized bronchodilators can be allowed two to three hours to achieve an effect, and if a satisfactory response is achieved then they can be repeated at intervals until the attack settles. If the attack is moderately severe or a mild exacerbation does not improve, or gets worse despite the equivalent of 5 mg salbutamol, then corticosteroids should be given. Some would argue that any patient with an exacerbation requiring high-dose inhaled bronchodilators should be given corticosteroids. All patients at risk should be taking inhaled corticosteroids.

The exact dose of corticosteroid and its route are not firmly established but as soon as possible the patient should receive a high loading oral dose of prednisolone as discussed previously. If the patient cannot swallow tablets and the attack is severe, a loading intravenous dose of hydrocortisone hemisuccinate should be given. A dose of 200 mg will be sufficient for most patients and this can be repeated on three or four occasions throughout the twenty-four hours, limiting the daily dose to about 1 g. Oral prednisolone should be started as soon as the patient can manage it, and intravenous hydrocortisone can be stopped twelve to twenty-four hours after the prednisolone has been given.

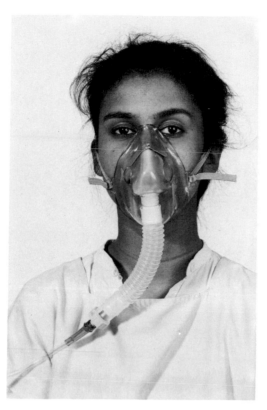

Figure 4.6 Hypoxia is a prominent feature of acute attacks of asthma and oxygen can be given freely. In chronic bronchitis and emphysema, carbon dioxide retention may occur. In such cases oxygen should be given in a controlled fashion and blood gases checked.

As already mentioned, it is always best to err on the side of giving steroids. If you feel it necessary to send the patient into hospital for further treatment it is very helpful to give a loading dose of intravenous or oral steroid before he or she leaves home.

Other measures

Fluids Those with a prolonged attack of severe asthma may become dehydrated through hyperventilation and difficulty in drinking. Although this is not a major problem in most patients, it is worth remembering to make sure the patient drinks fluid to avoid dehydration complicating recovery.

Oxygen If facilities exist at home or in the ambulance, oxygen therapy is best given. Only if the patient has chronic obstructive bronchitis is it necessary to use a low oxygen Ventimask such as a 24 per cent mask. Usually unlimited face-mask oxygen can be provided for the patient with asthma during a severe attack (Fig. 4.6).

There is a potential danger that bronchodilator therapy can increase hypoxia. It is not usually practical to give nebulizers with oxygen at home but it is advisable to administer oxygen to asthmatics in between nebulizations. This can be done with conventional oxygen apparatus.

ACUTE SEVERE ASTHMA IN ADULTS

Features of acute severe asthma

- Cannot complete sentences in one breath
- Respirations $\geq$ 25 breaths/min
- Pulse $\geq$110 beats/min
- Peak expiratory flow (PEF) $\leq$50% of predicted or best

Life-threatening features

- PEF <33% of predicted or best
- Silent chest, cyanosis, or feeble respiratory effort
- Bradycardia or hypotension
- Exhaustion, confusion, or coma

Markers of a very severe, life-threatening attack:

- Normal (5–6 kPa, 36–45 mm Hg) or high $PaCO_2$
- Severe hypoxia: PaO_2 <8 kPa (60 mm Hg) irrespective of treatment with oxygen
- A low pH (or high H^+)

Caution:

Patients with severe or life-threatening attacks may not be distressed and may not have all these abnormalities. The presence of any should alert the doctor.

Monitoring treatment

- Repeat measurement of PEF 15–30 minutes after starting treatment
- Oximetry: maintain SaO_2 >92%
- Repeat blood gas measurements within 2 hours of starting treatment if
  - initial PaO_2 <8 kPa (60 mmHg) unless subsequent SaO_2 >92%
  - $PaCO_2$ was normal or raised
  - patient deteriorates
- Chart PEF before and after giving nebulized or inhaled beta$_2$ agonists and at least 4 times daily throughout hospital stay
- Measure blood gases if SaO_2<92%

Treatment

- Oxygen – 40–60% (CO_2 retention is not aggravated by oxygen therapy in asthma)
- Salbutamol 5 mg or terbutaline 10 mg via an oxygen-driven nebulizer
- Prednisolone tablets 30–60 mg or intravenous hydrocortisone 200 mg, or both, if very ill
- No sedatives of any kind
- Chest radiograph to exclude pneumothorax

+ If life-threatening features are present:

- Add ipratropium 0.5 mg to the nebulized beta$_2$ agonist
- Give intravenous aminophylline 250 mg over 20 minutes or salbutamol or terbutaline 250 μg over 10 minutes. Do not give bolus aminophylline to patients already taking oral theophyllines

When discharged from hospital patients should have:

- Been on discharge medication for 24 hours and have had inhaler technique checked and recorded
- PEF >75% of predicted or best and PEF diurnal variability <25% unless discharge is agreed with respiratory physician
- Treatment with oral and inhaled steroid in addition to bronchodilators
- Own PEF meter and written self-management plan
- GP follow-up arranged within 1 week
- Follow-up appointment in respiratory clinic within 4 weeks

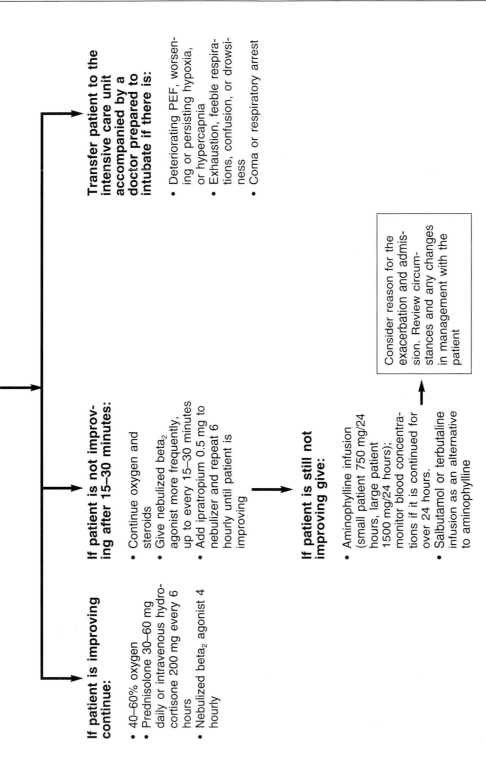

Transfer patient to the intensive care unit accompanied by a doctor prepared to intubate if there is:

- Deteriorating PEF, worsening or persisting hypoxia, or hypercapnia
- Exhaustion, feeble respirations, confusion, or drowsiness
- Coma or respiratory arrest

If patient is not improving after 15–30 minutes:

- Continue oxygen and steroids
- Give nebulized beta$_2$ agonist more frequently, up to every 15–30 minutes
- Add ipratropium 0.5 mg to nebulizer and repeat 6 hourly until patient is improving

If patient is still not improving give:

- Aminophylline infusion (small patient 750 mg/24 hours, large patient 1500 mg/24 hours); monitor blood concentrations if it is continued for over 24 hours.
- Salbutamol or terbutaline infusion as an alternative to aminophylline

Consider reason for the exacerbation and admission. Review circumstances and any changes in management with the patient

If patient is improving continue:

- 40–60% oxygen
- Prednisolone 30–60 mg daily or intravenous hydrocortisone 200 mg every 6 hours
- Nebulized beta$_2$ agonist 4 hourly

Figure 4.7 Guidelines for the treatment of acute severe asthma in adults. (Adapted with permission from the British Thoracic Society Guidelines[57])

ACUTE SEVERE ASTHMA IN ADULTS IN GENERAL PRACTICE

Regard each emergency consultation as for acute severe asthma until it is shown otherwise.

Assess and record:
• Symptoms and response to self-treatment
• Heart and respiratory rates
• Peak expiratory flow (PEF)

Caution:
Patients with severe or life-threatening attacks may not be distressed and may not have all these abnormalities. The presence of any should alert the doctor.

ASSESSMENT

Uncontrolled asthma

• Speech normal
• Pulse <110 beats/min
• Respiration <25 breaths/min
• PEF >50% predicted or best

Management
Treat at home but response to treatment MUST be assessed before you leave

Acute severe asthma

• Cannot complete sentences
• Pulse ≥110 beats/min
• Respiration ≥25 breaths/min
• PEF ≤50% of predicted or best

Management
Seriously consider admission if more than one feature above present

Life-threatening asthma

• Silent chest
• Cyanosis
• Bradycardia or exhaustion
• PEF <33% of predicted or best

Management
Arrange immediate ADMISSION

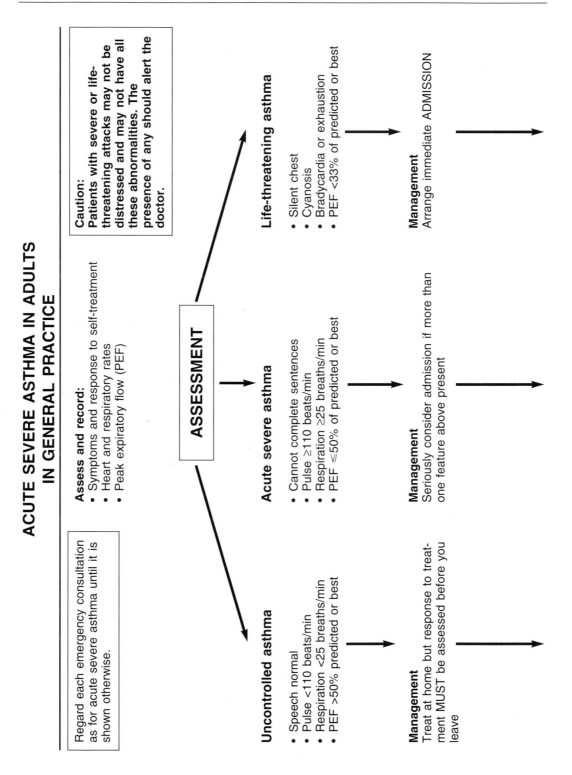

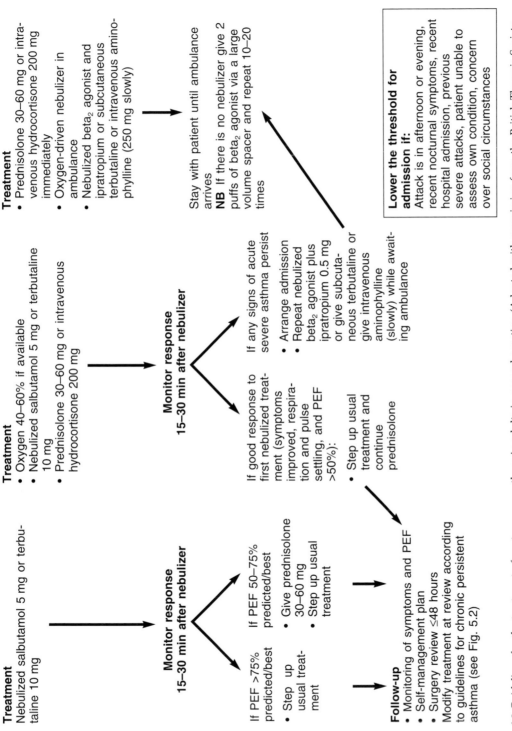

Treatment
Nebulized salbutamol 5 mg or terbutaline 10 mg

Monitor response 15–30 min after nebulizer

If PEF >75% predicted/best
• Step up usual treatment

If PEF 50–75% predicted/best
• Give prednisolone 30–60 mg
• Step up usual treatment

Follow-up
• Monitoring of symptoms and PEF
• Self-management plan
• Surgery review ≤48 hours
Modify treatment at review according to guidelines for chronic persistent asthma (see Fig. 5.2)

Treatment
• Oxygen 40–60% if available
• Nebulized salbutamol 5 mg or terbutaline 10 mg
• Prednisolone 30–60 mg or intravenous hydrocortisone 200 mg

Monitor response 15–30 min after nebulizer

If good response to first nebulized treatment (symptoms improved, respiration and pulse settling, and PEF >50%):
• Step up usual treatment and continue prednisolone

If any signs of acute severe asthma persist
• Arrange admission
• Repeat nebulized beta₂ agonist plus ipratropium 0.5 mg or give subcutaneous terbutaline or give intravenous aminophylline (slowly) while awaiting ambulance

Treatment
• Prednisolone 30–60 mg or intravenous hydrocortisone 200 mg immediately
• Oxygen-driven nebulizer in ambulance
• Nebulized beta₂ agonist and ipratropium or subcutaneous terbutaline or intravenous aminophylline (250 mg slowly)

Stay with patient until ambulance arrives
NB If there is no nebulizer give 2 puffs of beta₂ agonist via a large volume spacer and repeat 10–20 times

Lower the threshold for admission if:
Attack is in afternoon or evening, recent nocturnal symptoms, recent hospital admission, previous severe attacks, patient unable to assess own condition, concern over social circumstances

Figure 4.8 Guidelines for the treatment of acute severe asthma in adults in general practice. (Adapted with permission from the British Thoracic Society Guidelines.[57])

Sedation Whereas oxygen-induced respiratory depression is not usually a problem with asthma itself, the use of sedatives can be very dangerous. Asthmatic patients breathe with every muscle in their body and sometimes are very sensitive to respiratory depressants. These can include such apparently safe drugs as temazepam and diazepam; thus all sedation is best avoided. The best way to reduce anxiety associated with the attack is to treat the attack itself.

Antibiotics are only required if there is good evidence for infection. As a general rule antibiotics have little effect on outcome and should only play a subsidiary role in the treatment of acute asthma. Even when exacerbations of asthma appear to be precipitated by infection, the causative organism is usually a virus and not susceptible to antibiotic treatment.[33]

HOME OR HOSPITAL?

Most attacks of asthma respond rapidly to an increase in the treatment, only a few being severe enough to warrant admission to hospital (guidelines for the management of these patients have been adapted from the British Thoracic Society Guidelines[57] (Fig. 4.7)). Most patients have sufficiently predictable asthmatic attacks for you to plan with them their response, but a few unfortunately are liable to fulminant attacks which can be life-threatening. These can arise with ferocious rapidity, making rapid access to hospital essential. This requires the full cooperation of patient and local hospital as well as the practitioner. Rare at-risk patients need to be identified in advance and the best mechanism for rapid access has to be preplanned at local level.

All asthmatic patients and their close relatives must be aware of precisely what to do in an acute attack. They must know what therapy to take and where they should seek further help. Again, all this should be carefully planned beforehand and incorporated into a written action plan and a self-management strategy.

At-risk patients

These not only include those with a history of acute fulminant attacks but also patients who have been admitted previously for severe asthma and those requiring repeated courses of prednisolone. Patients displaying marked circadian rhythmicity with sleep disturbance are also at risk, as are those patients whose lung function is gradually but remorselessly deteriorating.

EDUCATING THE PATIENT

In these at-risk groups as well as with other patients, it is best to agree with the patient what index of worsening of their asthma should lead to a change in management.

This can be seen in Fig. 4.8. where indices of asthma severity are listed. Where peak flow can be measured this can be used to guide medication but clinical indices are also important. Increasing use of inhaled beta$_2$ agonists plus sleep disturbance are important factors in loss of asthma control. Criteria for asthma control are discussed further in the next chapter.

PRACTICAL POINTS

- The majority of the problems in acute attacks of asthma come from under-treatment, rather than overtreatment. Appropriate early therapy to prevent deterioration is much simpler than trying to rescue an asthmatic from a severe attack.
- The main features of the treatment are increased doses of beta$_2$ agonists, possibly by nebulizer, and administration of corticosteroids.
- When using aminophylline the initial injection must be given slowly and reduced if oral theophylline are being used.
- In severe attacks it is helpful to be able to administer oxygen at home while awaiting transfer to hospital.
- All sedation should be avoided.
- A vital part of the management is to educate the patient as to when and how to seek further help.
- Patients should plan a self-management strategy and criteria for good asthma control with the help of their physicians.

5
Management of chronic asthma

BACKGROUND

The management of patients with asthma depends on the frequency of attacks, their severity and the possibility of their avoidance. Infrequent attacks can largely be managed by treating the attack when it arises but if the frequency increases then it becomes more necessary to take pre-emptive action to suppress the asthmatic attacks. It is difficult to be precise about the exact frequency demanding suppressive therapy but, in general, attacks occurring more frequently than one per month are best dealt with by chronic regular treatment, whereas attacks occurring only three or four times per annum can usually be treated on an *ad hoc* basis. Between these frequencies, much depends upon the severity of the attacks and the patient's attitude towards them. The treatment of each attack when it occurs will again depend upon its severity and may require a high-dose course of prednisolone on the one hand or a couple of puffs of bronchodilator aerosol on the other.

Treatment for chronic asthma is now influenced by recently drawn up guidelines or consensus statements. These are based on criteria for control of asthma which are now more stringent than in the past. A number of criteria for control of asthma have been proposed; a practical list is shown in the table below:

- prevent chronic and troublesome symptoms (eg cough and breathlessness)
- maintain (near) normal pulmonary function
- maintain daily variation in PEF <10%
- maintain normal activity levels, including exercise
- prevent exacerbations
- provide optimal pharmacotherapy with minimal or no adverse effects
- meet patients' and families' expectations of and satisfaction with asthma care

How best to achieve asthma control requires a comprehensive programme as set out in the NIH International Consensus Report[58] as follows:

Asthma management has six interrelated parts:
1. Educate patients to develop a partnership in asthma management
2. Assess and monitor asthma severity with objective measures of lung function
3. Avoid or control asthma triggers

4. Establish medication plans for chronic management
5. Establish plans for managing exacerbations
6. Provide regular follow-up care

This chapter is mainly devoted to medication for chronic asthma and divides medication into those for relief of symptoms, e.g. inhaled beta$_2$ agonists, and those to prevent or control or suppress symptoms, e.g. inhaled corticosteroids.

ENVIRONMENTAL CONTROL

As with other conditions it is best to avoid attacks if this is possible but unfortunately this state of affairs is unusual in asthma.

Avoidance of precipitating factors

Many asthmatics are atopic but only a few clearly identify a cause for their asthma and even fewer find it easy to avoid this cause.

Avoidable causes include hazards related to specific occupations (see Chapter 3) but many patients find it difficult to give up work and have to rely on work practices being changed or the availability of other jobs within the organization that do not expose them to the sensitizing agent.

The other common avoidable causes of asthma are usually of a recreational nature, such as horse riding or owning a pet (see Chapter 3). Once again, many asthmatic patients prefer to continue with their recreation and cope with the asthma it produces rather than give up the recreation.

Where the house dust mite plays an important role in the genesis of asthma, scrupulous attention to house dust control and the dispersal of the mite from mattresses, blankets and pillows is either seldom successful or beyond the patience and diligence of most asthmatic sufferers and their families.

Growing evidence of the importance of indoor aeroallergens both in inducing asthma in children and in triggering attacks, has led to increasing research into environmental control. These include enclosing bedding in impermeable sheets and pillows, better indoor ventilation and dehumidification. If successful these measures might limit the increase in prevalence of childhood asthma as well as reduce the need for medication. As yet it is not possible to assess the value of these measures which require more research to establish their role.

Moving into hospital has been shown to help some patients with asthma,[35] as they thereby avoid the allergens in their home, but this is hardly a practical course of action. Neither is the policy of moving children to holiday homes or schools at high altitude. The basis for any success from such a move may be related to removal from emotional stress as well as the avoidance of allergens.

Desensitization

In Chapter 8 the role of desensitization (immunotherapy) will be discussed as another way of preventing asthma arising in patients sensitized to an identifiable allergen. At this stage suffice it to say that this approach is only likely to be successful in those few patients with pure grass pollen asthma, although some success has also been claimed for house mite desensitization.[36] The improvements gained are usually marginal and may be associated with a significant morbidity. Control is more effectively achieved with simple pharmacological therapy.[60] Desensitization needs to be repeated yearly and has not been shown to be of any value to allergens other than pollen, rag weed and probably cats, as well as house dust mite.[37] Therefore the practice of making up a cocktail of desensitization injections based on the results of positive skin testing is a triumph of hope over scientific evidence.

There is general agreement that immunotherapy for asthma should only be employed if medication is not effective or suitable. It should not be given to patients with moderate or severe asthma in view of the risks of fatal anaphylaxis. If given, full resuscitation facilities are required.

WHICH TYPE OF TREATMENT?

The poor overall success rate of environmental control and desensitization to date means that the majority of management is based on drug therapy. That is not to dismiss all other non-pharmacological measures, but in general these are only of marginal or occasional value and seldom have a substantial scientific foundation. Treatments such as acupuncture involve a large placebo component.[61]

Relaxation therapy and hypnotherapy have been demonstrated occasionally to improve asthma control, but when used on a regular basis have proved disappointing in practice[62] (see Chapter 10). Likewise, behavioural therapy may occasionally appear to work but the resources required for this are considerable and there is no evidence that used on a widespread scale it compares favourably with effective drug therapy.

In contrast, drug therapy is highly effective in the majority of patients, is easy to use and is sufficiently safe to provide the basic management of patients with asthma. With the possible exception of theophylline, the drugs currently available are safer than asthma itself and their use over the past decade or so has improved the lives of many asthmatics who, being disabled for much of the time, were previously unable to lead anything like a normal existence.

MANAGEMENT STRATEGY

Treat attacks vigorously

Attacks are generally best treated by intensive therapy as it is better to overtreat than undertreat at this stage. When an asthmatic develops an acute attack it is best to treat this with as high a dose as possible rather than take too timid an approach. Of course, as when treating other conditions, it is also important to try and find the minimum dose necessary to control symptoms. Rapid high-dose treatment will quickly abolish the asthmatic attack, whereas cautious increases in dose may only chase the symptoms as they deteriorate, leaving the patient on a high-dose treatment but still with asthma. The reasons for this are not clear and this view is based on general experience; most patients who have experienced both approaches will readily testify to the success of vigorous treatment. Patients usually soon learn which attacks are best treated by a minor increase in their existing therapy and which circumstances suggest that an attack needs to be treated more intensively.

In general, the need to use intensive and aggressive therapy for an attack is increased if the patient has poor lung function or a history of recurrent severe attacks requiring hospital admission. Thus, in a patient with stable asthma and a nearly normal peak flow, an attack is likely to be best treated by increasing the dose of treatment. On the other hand, in a patient who is on steroids and who has a history of previous hospital admissions, an attack with a very low peak flow is best given the benefit of the doubt and treated much more intensively.

These considerations were encapsulated into recommendations by the British Thoracic Society in 1990 as shown below:[57]

Treatment with short course of steroids

Short courses of steroids may be needed to control exacerbations of asthma at any step. Indications are:

- Symptoms and peak expiratory flow get progressively worse each day
- Peak expiratory flow falls below 60% of patient's best result
- Sleep is disturbed by asthma
- Morning symptoms persist until midday
- Maximum treatment not including oral steroids does not work
- Emergency nebulizer or injected bronchodilators are needed

Give patients prednisolone 30–60 mg daily (60 mg if they are already taking oral steroids) until two days after full recovery, with symptoms resolved and peak flow up to 80% of patient's best, when the drug may be stopped or the dose tapered.

If arranged beforehand short courses of oral steroids may be started on the patient's initiative according to written guidance.

Prophylactic suppressive therapy

Prevention or control   Traditionally, asthma is treated on the basis of symptoms and therefore therapy is usually attack related. As mentioned above, this is a reasonable policy if the attacks are intermittent and sporadic, but if they occur more frequently and follow a fairly predictable pattern then it is worth considering taking pre-emptive action by suppressing the underlying causes of asthma. These causes are not only external ones, such as sensitizing agents, but constitutional factors.

Bronchial hyperresponsiveness   In addition to a genetic predisposition, bronchial hyperresponsiveness is probably the other most important pathogenic mechanism underlying asthma. This renders the airways abnormally sensitive to stimuli and this can readily be demonstrated in patients by inhaling agents such as histamine or cold air. The airway irritability subserves exercise-induced asthma and the wheezing produced by laughter and yawning.

Airway reactivity also plays an important role in exaggerating the normal circadian rhythmicity in lung function. Airway size varies over a twenty-four hour cycle, being widest during the day and narrower at night.[63] Even in healthy subjects, small fluctuations in peak flow can be demonstrated, but in asthma these rhythmic changes are much greater, with the patient having a lower mean peak flow and a much larger amplitude of peak flow variation. The highest values are usually in the afternoon with the lowest peak flow at about 4.00 am. These circadian fluctuations account for the clinical features of sleep disturbance and the fact that asthmatic patients are usually worse when they wake up in the morning.

Nocturnal asthma   Often responds to the usual asthmatic treatments aimed at generally reducing airway reactivity throughout the day. Where it remains a particular problem, the use of long-acting drugs, such as slow-release oral beta$_2$ agonists or slow-release theophylline, last thing at night, may be helpful.

Recently long-acting inhaled beta$_2$ agonists such as salmeterol and formoterol have been used to control nocturnal asthma. They are particularly useful in patients who have sleep disturbance while taking anti-inflammatory medication, replacing the oral alternatives.

Reducing airway hyperresponsiveness   Bronchial hyperresponsiveness is an important pathogenic mechanism to which therapy should be directed. At present we have relatively little knowledge of the effects of asthma therapies on bronchial reactivity but there is evidence that most asthma treatments can modify it. A reduction in bronchial reactivity has been shown following inhalation of selective beta$_2$ agonists, which may account for their distinctive success in preventing exercise-induced asthma.

Anti-inflammatory treatment can reduce bronchial hyperresponsiveness and the best results are achieved by inhaled corticosteroids.[64] Although very effective, inhaled corticosteroids seldom are able to restore hyperresponsive airways back to normal.

The importance of bronchial reactivity leads to a valuable strategic principle, namely to treat bronchial reactivity continuously, thereby limiting asthma attacks, rather than to wait until the attacks arise before treating them. Unless the attacks are sporadic, we believe treatment to suppress via anti-inflammatory medication has much to commend it and this view is now supported by guideline recommendations.

Increased safety of inhaled therapy   The use of regular suppressive or preventive treatment for asthma depends to a large extent upon the treatment being safe and effective. Over the last decade or so the pharmacological agents have been refined to be more selective and the increased use of inhaled therapy has enabled the dose delivered to be much reduced, thereby enhancing the safety margin of treatment. Regular inhaled therapy to suppress asthma appears to be safer than poorly controlled airway irritability and regular asthmatic attacks. Clinical trials have demonstrated the effectiveness and safety of inhaled steroids in controlling asthma over long periods[65,66]

ROUTE OF ADMINISTRATION

It is important at this stage to review why inhaled therapy is best used as the standard method for drug delivery in the majority of patients with asthma. The merits can be simply stated: inhaled therapy enables a small dose of effective treatment to be delivered direct to the airway. This minimizes the risk of side-effects both by reducing the dose as well as the need for the drug to reach the target organ via the circulation.

This can be best seen by way of example. Most asthma patients respond well to a selective beta$_2$ agonist such as salbutamol. Effective bronchodilatation can be achieved by both the oral and the inhaled route, with 4 mg (4,000 mcg) by mouth being equivalent to 200 mcg by aerosol. Thus the same degree of bronchial dilatation is achieved by the inhaled route using a dose one-twentieth that of the oral route. It is not surprising that systemic side-effects are much less likely using the hand-held inhaler.

The same consideration applies with even greater force to the use of corticosteroids. The standard dose of inhaled beclomethasone dipropionate of 400 mcg is equivalent to between 5 and 10 mg daily of prednisolone, and yet the risks of systemic side-effects are only found in the patients taking prednisolone (see pages 52 and 118).

Oral therapy and other routes of administration are therefore no more effective and are likely to produce adverse systemic side-effects. Systemic side-effects are a particular problem with theophylline, which is an effective bronchodilator but which unfortunately cannot be taken by inhalation.

Theophylline causes a wide range of systemic side-effects and is much less selective than the beta$_2$ agonists in common use. In addition to gastrointestinal side-effects it produces cardiac and neurotoxicity, and unfortunately can produce fatalities.[67] This can arise from oral use as well as following intravenous therapy in the acutely ill asthmatic. One of the basic reasons for this unpredictability is that patients vary considerably in the way they metabolize theophylline and therefore it is very difficult to predict a blood level achieved by any oral dose. To avoid toxic levels and yet ensure therapeutic blood levels, it is advisable to monitor blood levels of theophylline to establish the appropriate oral dose for each patient.

Blood level monitoring is essential when giving intravenous aminophylline to patients, particularly if they are already on sustained-release xanthine preparations, or are sick with heart failure, renal disease or hepatic insufficiency (see pages 53 and 117). As theophylline therapy is not significantly more effective than beta$_2$ agonist or other bronchodilator treatment, its use should be reserved for those patients not responding to inhaled bronchodilators, as the risks associated with its use are significant. In practice, theophylline will only occasionally be required, as the majority of patients can be treated satisfactorily with inhaled beta$_2$ agonists or inhaled anticholinergics.

The best route of administration

In summary, most patients can be treated satisfactorily with inhaled treatment, which can consist of bronchodilators, sodium cromoglycate or steroids. This provides an adequate range of treatment for acute attacks and suppression, and by using the inhaled route the safety margin of treatment is much better than other routes of administration.

Leukotriene antagonists need to be taken orally. In some cases absorption is affected by food; the leukotriene receptor antagonist zafirlukast must be taken an hour before or two hours after meals.

ASTHMA GUIDELINES

Before considering the medication available to control and prevent asthma it is best to see how the individual treatments fit into an overall plan for management of chronic asthma. Guidelines have been drawn up for this purpose based on:

1. The criteria for control of asthma
2. A stepwise approach based on treatment related to severity.
3. Patient education

Asthma severity is based on symptoms, use of relief medication and where possible measurements of lung function, usually peak expiratory flow. Bronchodilators are used primarily to resolve symptoms, and their use is thus an index of severity. Long-acting bronchodilators by inhalation or orally can protect against symptoms, particularly at night, but should not be used as primary preventive medication as their clinical non-bronchodilating properties remain to be evaluated. Therefore, inhaled anti-inflammatory medication is the treatment of choice for chronic asthma. Charts from the latest British Thoracic Society Guidelines (1995/7) are shown on pages 74–5 and 88–9 to demonstrate the current consensus in the UK concerning the management of chronic asthma in adults and children. Although the guidelines show a series of steps it is best to try to achieve control as soon as possible by choosing a suitable entry step and cutting back treatment to a maintenance level once adequate control has been established.

BRONCHODILATOR THERAPY

Bronchodilators provide treatment for symptom relief. They can be used to treat acute episodes and all patients will probably require an aerosol containing a short-acting selective beta$_2$ agonist to deal with the acute attack. There is general agreement that this is the best treatment as, unlike oral therapy, the inhaled route not only minimizes systemic side-effects but also produces a very rapid onset of action.

Regular use

Over the past few years, it has become clear that bronchodilators may have properties other than that of bronchodilation. These appear to include blocking specific and nonspecific challenge, the inhibition of mediator release, as well as stimulation of mucociliary clearance. These additional properties may help deal with the inflammatory component of asthma and may provide grounds for using bronchodilators on a regular basis to suppress asthma. This view is countered by evidence that regular treatment with beta$_2$ agonists may impair control of asthma.[68] On the other hand, studies with long-acting salmeterol have shown better control of asthma.[69] In mild persistent asthma a comparison of regular and intermittent use of a short acting β agonist showed no significant differences and concluded that there was no advantage or clinically important disadvantage in regular use.[70] Recent guidelines place salmeterol with low to medium dose inhaled steroids (<1000 mcg beclomethasone dipropionate or budesonide) as an alternative to higher dose inhaled steroids.

Inhaled or oral?

The advantages of inhaled therapy would suggest that when given on a regular basis, bronchodilators should still be taken by inhalation; however, some clinicians prefer to use oral therapy on a twice-daily basis using slow-release preparations, as this may improve patient adherence to therapy. In a symptomatic disease like asthma there is no evidence that compliance is improved by decreased frequency of administration.[71] This potential advantage also has to be set against the problems of systemic side-effects and the fact that most patients need inhaled bronchodilators only two or three times a day to achieve a satisfactory result.

Problems with inhalers

The two main problems associated with inhaled therapy are:

1. The fear that inhalers may have been associated with the epidemic of death in the 1960s and more recently in New Zealand in the 1970s.
2. The difficulties some patients have with manipulating aerosols.

Fear of inhalers   This appears to be ill founded. With the introduction of salbutamol in 1969 and other more selective beta$_2$ agonists since then, the use of inhalers has grown considerably and is now well in excess of levels in the mid-1960s – but there has not been a return of the epidemic other than in New Zealand. As we mentioned previously, the use of inhalers before death is much more likely to be a sign that asthma is deteriorating than that their use is implicated in the mortality. In retrospect it is likely that it was asthma that killed most patients during the epidemic, the inhaler usage merely indicating the need for further treatment. This view has been supported by the recent meta-analysis report.[23]

Difficulty with inhaler delivery systems   The major problem with inhaled therapy concerns the delivery system. Pressurized aerosols are in widespread use and prove to be convenient and effective, but unfortunately 20 per cent of patients cannot use them appropriately. The main problem is one of synchronization, but other errors occur, such as failure to hold the breath following inhalation of bronchodilator. This occurs even when care is taken to teach patients how to use an inhaler. Although not always successful, educating patients on correct inhaler technique will undoubtedly reduce the scale of the problem (see Chapter 9).

New easy-to-use inhalers   In face of these difficulties, other delivery systems have been introduced and more are being planned. These range from small hand-held devices such as the Accuhaler, Autohaler or Turbohaler to nebulizer and spacer devices such as the Nebuhaler, Babyhaler and Volumatic (see Chapter 9).

Powder delivery systems such as the Diskhaler, Diskus/Accuhaler and Turbohaler are useful because they avoid the problem of synchronization, the device being actuated by the act of inspiration. Furthermore, they are small and convenient, and have proved to be of great value in the treatment of children with asthma. They also enable the clinician to differentiate clearly for patients between the inhalers for regular suppressive therapy, and the pressurized aerosol for emergency use. They can be left by the bedside to be used night and morning which clearly identifies that treatment is different from the pressurized inhaler of salbutamol which is carried with the patient in case of an acute episode. This helps overcome the confusion that often arises in the minds of patients as to which treatment is to be used for attacks and which for their prevention.

Nebulizers

These are being increasingly used and they probably have two advantages:

1. The first is not peculiar to nebulizers but stems from the fact that the respirator solution contains a much higher dose of beta$_2$ agonist or steroid and therefore nebulized therapy delivers a much larger dose. Such an increase could of course be achieved by increasing the number of inhalations of a hand-held metered dose or powder inhaler.

2. Breathing a mist of bronchodilator or steroid enhances drug delivery, as synchronization is not required.

The latter problem is also overcome by the use of devices such as a powder delivery inhaler and therefore the actual merits of using the nebulizer in preference to high doses of a patient-actuated inhaler are not established.

Unfortunately, many patients acquire a nebulizer and use it almost indiscriminately. As the dose thus taken can mount rapidly this may lead to a further public worry if death occurs under these circumstances. As with the inhalers in the 1960s and 1970s, the high dose of bronchodilator may obscure the need for extra treatment and nebulizers may be blamed for deaths when in fact the severity of the asthma and the need for extra treatment were not recognized. Patients should be warned about this. Nebulizer therapy must be very carefully supervised and if the patient uses it excessively extra treatment must be provided.

Spacers

The other improvement in delivery system has been the introduction in the 1980s of extension tubes and spacers. These improve the delivery of respirable particles of drugs and will be discussed along with the other delivery systems in Chapter 9. At this point, suffice to say that over the next few years many new delivery systems are likely to be introduced, improving the prospects for inhaled therapy being available for the majority of patients.

Selective beta$_2$ agonists

Since the introduction of salbutamol in 1969, many other selective beta$_2$ agonists have appeared on the market but there is very little to choose between them as they have similar actions to salbutamol. These agents are still to be preferred over the less selective adrenergic agents such as isoprenaline or adrenaline, their selectivity of action and suitability for use as inhaled therapy having provided effective and safe bronchodilator treatment over the past decade and a half.

Anticholinergic agents

The use of anticholinergic drugs in the treatment of asthma goes back beyond the turn of the century but atropinic treatment fell out of favour because of side-effects and the

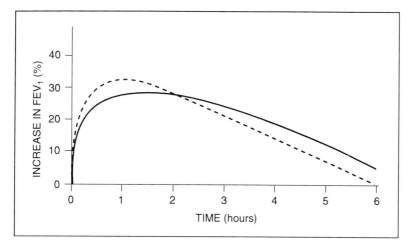

Figure 5.1 Typical bronchodilator responses to salbutamol (---) and ipratropium bromide (—) in asthma. The time to peak action is slower for ipratropium but the effect is more prolonged.

fear that it dried airway secretions, possibly promoting mucus plugging. The introduction of ipratropium bromide in the mid-1970s has revived interest in this treatment as it can provide effective bronchodilatation with few side-effects (Fig. 5.1). It has also been shown not to adversely effect sputum or mucociliary clearance, and when used in combination with a beta$_2$ agonist below maximally effective dose has an additive effect. Ipratropium bromide can be of value for patients not responding well to selective beta$_2$ agonists and it appears to be more successful in older patients rather than in young adults or children, where selective beta$_2$ agonists are more likely to be successful.

Ipratropium bromide can be used both for treating acute attacks and for maintenance therapy, and plays a valuable role supplementing the use of selective beta$_2$ agonists, particularly in the more elderly asthma patient. Oxitropium bromide is similar but has a longer duration of action.

Theophylline

Some of the problems with theophylline therapy have been discussed above and in the previous chapter. They should not obscure the fact that methyl xanthines such as theophylline can provide effective treatment and are in widespread use throughout the world. New sustained-release preparations have enabled the drug to be taken once or twice a day, which is undoubtedly more convenient for patients; and if it were not for the toxic nature of its side-effects theophylline might have a much greater role in the management of asthma.

Unfortunately it is the only commonly used asthma drug which may cause death and as it is not significantly better as a bronchodilator than the other agents, its use should be reserved for patients not responding to the full available range of inhaled therapy, or for the occasional patient who cannot or will not use inhalers.

Used intelligently as recommended in the guidelines, theophylline can play a very useful role but its potentially hazardous side-effects make it an unlikely candidate for first-line bronchodilator therapy as most patients can be treated perfectly adequately with other drugs.

When a patient requires theophylline, it is probably best to use a sustained-release preparation, but it is equally important to judge the correct dose by having the plasma theophylline measured in a laboratory. Once this dose has been calculated, then repeated measurements of theophylline levels are rarely required unless a change occurs in the patient, such as giving up smoking, or, in a child, acquiring an acute respiratory illness (see page 117).

Recent work suggests that at lower doses than usually required for bronchodilating airways, theophylline may have immunomodulating and anti-inflammatory properties. The clinical significance of these observations requires evaluation.

SODIUM CROMOGLYCATE

When sodium cromoglycate was introduced in 1967, it was correctly perceived as an important new drug. It provided effective treatment for asthma and appeared to act directly on an important pathogenic mechanism, namely mediator release. At the time of its introduction, patients – especially children – were either having to take increasing doses of isoprenaline to control their asthma, which produced cardiac side-effects, or were forced to take systemic corticosteroids, which in children often stunted growth. Sodium cromoglycate provided a very useful bridge between these two courses of action, enabling the dose of isoprenaline to be kept down and averting the need for systemic corticosteroids in many patients.

Sodium cromoglycate remains a valuable drug, fulfilling the same original role but its use has been diminished by recent developments. Firstly, selective beta$_2$ agonists have enabled bronchodilators to be used in higher doses without adverse side-effects. Furthermore, the introduction of inhaled corticosteroids has improved the prospect for steroid therapy, enabling it to be used more frequently than prednisolone or ACTH, and further narrowing the therapeutic role for sodium cromoglycate.

Its use today

Although originally produced to be taken as a powder, using a Spinhaler, a metered dose inhaler is also available which provides a greater range of options for patient use (see Chapter 9). The role of sodium cromoglycate in controlling bronchial hyperresponsiveness has been identified but its precise mode of action has become more controversial as it may not act primarily on mediator release and at present there is some argument as to how sodium cromoglycate achieves its beneficial results.[72]

Sodium cromoglycate can be used on a regular basis to suppress asthma, particularly in children when the asthma is of allergic origin. It may also be used before exercise or allergen challenge to prevent asthma but this is less commonly an indication because inhaled beta$_2$ agonists are usually more successful in preventing attacks and are of especial value in treating exercise-induced asthma.

The role of sodium cromoglycate has been emphasised by the importance given to anti-inflammatory medication by asthma guidelines. The absence of adverse side-effects makes sodium cromoglycate an alternative to inhaled corticosteroids in controlling chronic childhood asthma although it is often thought to be not as efficacious.[73]

NEDOCROMIL SODIUM

Nedocromil sodium has a very similar role to that of sodium cromoglycate. It also probably has anti-inflammatory properties and can be used as medication for controlling asthma. Its safety profile is not as well known as sodium cromoglycate and its comparable efficacy has not been fully established.

Like sodium cromoglycate its role in asthma guidelines is in competition with inhaled corticosteroids for use as regular therapy for chronic asthma. The choice between these treatments will depend on judgement about comparisons of effectiveness, safety and cost-effectiveness.

CORTICOSTEROIDS

When corticosteroids were first assessed in the mid-1950s, there was some doubt about their effectiveness, but over the last thirty years there has been a universal acceptance that corticosteroids can effectively suppress asthma. They are particularly useful in aborting a deterioration in asthma control but are also very effective when taken on a regular basis.

When taken as a short oral course to treat an acute attack there are very few side-effects associated with systemic steroids, and drugs like prednisolone remain the treatment of choice for a severe acute attack of asthma not responding to bronchodilators. On the other hand, when systemic corticosteroids are taken on a regular basis to suppress asthma, side-effects are more likely and have proved to be a burden for many patients with damaging consequences. A small number of difficult asthmatics appear to be unresponsive to corticosteroids.

Inhaled steroids

The introduction of inhaled corticosteroids with the licensing of beclomethasone dipropionate (BDP) in 1972 has radically changed this situation. Inhaled BDP has provided effective steroid treatment for asthma without clinically adverse side-effects. Over the first twenty years' use of BDP, there have been no reported cases of Cushing's syndrome although some systemic activity can be detected by assessing hypothalamo–pituitary–adrenal (HPA) function. This activity becomes more likely at higher doses, but clinical side-effects are not observed at doses of up to 1.5–2.0 mg per day of BDP or its most recent equivalents.

When first introduced, inhaled steroids were used four times daily, but it has now been shown that morning and evening administration using the same total daily dose is just as effective.[74] Recent experience has also shown that higher doses produce greater

MANAGEMENT OF CHRONIC ASTHMA IN ADULTS AND SCHOOLCHILDREN

- Avoidance of provoking factors where possible
- Patient's involvement and education
- Selection of best inhaler device
- Treatment stepped up as necessary to achieve good control
- Treatment stepped down if control of asthma good

The expert panel report of the US National Heart, Lung and Blood Institute (NHLBI) in 1997 has similar steps except that the BTS steps 3 and 4 appear as two parts of step 3. The NHLBI report states that anti-leukotrienes may be considered as an alternative at step 2 although it cautions that further clinical experience and study are needed to establish the role of these agents in asthma therapy.[75]

Step 1:

Occasional use of relief bronchodilators

Inhaled short-acting β agonists 'as required' for symptom relief are acceptable. If they are needed more than once daily move to step 2.
Before altering a treatment step ensure that the patient is having the treatment and has a good inhaler technique. Address any fears.

Step 2:

Regular inhaled anti-inflammatory agents

Inhaled short-acting β agonists as required
plus:
beclomethasone or budesonide 100–400 µg twice daily or fluticasone 50–200 µg twice daily. Alternatively, use cromoglycate or nedocromil sodium, but if control is not achieved start inhaled steroids.

Step 3:

High-dose inhaled steroids or low dose inhaled steroids plus long acting inhaled β agonist bronchodilator

Inhaled short-acting β agonists as required
plus either:
beclomethasone or budesonide increased to 800–2000 µg daily or fluticasone 400–1000 µg daily via a large volume spacer
or:
beclomethasone or budesonide 100–400 µg twice daily or fluticasone 50–200 µg twice daily plus salmeterol 50 µg twice daily.
In a very small number of patients who experience side effects with high dose inhaled steroids, either the long acting inhaled β agonist option is used *or* a sustained release theophylline may be added to step 2 medication. Cromoglycate or nedocromil may also be tried.

Outcome of steps 1–3: control of asthma

- Minimal (ideally no) chronic symptoms, including nocturnal symptoms
- Minimal (infrequent) exacerbations
- Minimal need for relieving bronchodilators
- No limitations on activities including exercise
- Circadian variation in peak expiratory flow (PEF) <20%
- PEF ≥80% of predicted or best
- Minimal (or no) adverse effects from medicine

Figure 5.2 British Thoracic Society Guidelines on the management of chronic asthma in adults. (Reproduced with permission from ref. 57.)

Notes
- Patients should start treatment at the step most appropriate to the initial severity. A rescue course of prednisolone may be needed at any time and at any step. The aim is to achieve early control of the condition and then to reduce treatment.
- Until growth is complete any child requiring beclomethasone or budesonide > 800 μg daily or fluticasone >500 μg daily should be referred to a paediatrician with an interest in asthma.

Prescribe a peak flow meter and monitor response to treatment

Step 4:

High-dose inhaled steroids and regular bronchodilators

Inhaled short-acting β agonists as required with inhaled beclomethasone or budesonide 800–2000 μg daily or fluticasone 400–1000 μg daily via a large volume spacer
plus:
a sequential therapeutic trial of one or more of:
- inhaled long-acting β agonists
- sustained release theophylline
- inhaled ipratropium or oxitropium
- long-acting β agonist tablets
- high-dose inhaled bronchodilators
- cromoglycate or nedocromil

Step 5:

Addition of regular steroid tablets

Inhaled short-acting β agonists as required with inhaled beclomethasone or budesonide 800–2000 μg daily or fluticasone 400–1000 μg daily via a large volume spacer and one or more of the long acting bronchodilators
plus:
regular prednisolone tablets in a single daily dose

Stepping down

Review treatment every three to six months. If control is achieved a stepwise reduction in treatment may be possible. In patients whose treatment was recently started at step 4 or 5 or included steroid tablets for gaining control of asthma this reduction may take place after a short interval. In other patients with chronic asthma a three to six month period of stability should be shown before slow stepwise reduction is undertaken.

Outcome of steps 4 – 5: best possible results

- Least possible symptoms
- Least possible need for relieving bronchodilators
- Least possible limitation of activity
- Least possible variation in PEF
- Best PEF
- Least adverse effects from medicine

in association with the General Practitioner in Asthma Group, the British Association of Accident and Emergency Medicine, the British Paediatric Respiratory Society and the Royal College of Paediatrics and Child Health

benefit,[76] which might be expected from the results of prednisolone and ACTH treatment. Higher dose regimens are therefore more frequently used and, to assist this, preparations that give a higher dose per actuation have been introduced.

Other inhaled steroids

Since BDP was introduced over twenty years ago, many other clinically effective inhaled steroids have been introduced. These include flunisolide, triamcinolone acetonide, budesonide and fluticasone propionate. Fluticasone is effective at half the equivalent dose of BDP and budesonide. It is given as an alternative in the latest BTS recommendations. The relative systemic effects of the different inhaled corticosteroids are still under debate. Some studies in the literature are influenced by the different delivery devices used as well as the drug itself.

Indications

Because the experience gained with inhaled steroids showed them to be effective and because they had a wider safety margin than systemic treatment, clinicians began using inhaled steroids more freely than systemic ones such as prednisolone.

With growing confidence about their efficacy and safety, inhaled steroids have increasingly become the first choice of preventive therapy for chronic asthma in recent surveys of respiratory physicians. This important role as a key anti-inflammatory treatment for asthma has been incorporated into all guidelines and consensus reports. Clinical trials have demonstrated effectiveness in control of exacerbations with concurrent improvements in symptom control, lung function and bronchial hyperresponsiveness.[64,65,66] In doses up to 800–1,000 mcg per day inhaled steroids have acquired a good safety profile reputation and they are often regarded in these doses as the primary treatment for chronic asthma requiring daily use of bronchodilators.

Higher doses of inhaled steroids sometimes produce additional effectiveness, but this is not always the case. Many patients appear to benefit as much or more by adding a bronchodilator. Thus, inhaled steroids given twice daily at doses of up to 1 mg per day plus an inhaled long-acting inhaled beta$_2$ agonist also given twice daily have been included in some guidelines as alternatives to higher dose inhaled steroids as the next step when the asthma is severe enough to require more than 1 mg per day of inhaled steroid plus short-acting beta$_2$ agonists for breakthrough symptoms.[77,78] The addition of a long-acting bronchodilator is particularly useful for sleep disturbance. Further clinical trials will enable this course of action to be evaluated.

OTHER TREATMENTS

Although most patients can be treated adequately with inhaled bronchodilators and inhaled anti-inflammatory medication, there are other pharmacological agents available.

Antihistamines

Oral   H$_1$ blockers have been tried for many years and are often used in proprietary cough mixtures. There appears to be little evidence that this treatment benefits asthmatic patients, although the mild sedation may explain why patients and parents of children are sometimes happy with the effects of antihistamine-containing cough mixtures. Unfortunately sedation is a potentially dangerous side-effect as it may produce respiratory depression during acute attacks. Any benefits are more than outweighed by its risks.

Newer nonsedating antihistamines such as terfenadine and astemizole avoid these risks but their role in chronic asthma remains contentious.

Leukotriene antagonists

Oral inhibitors of leukotriene action may help to reduce the inflammatory component of asthma. Anti-leukotrienes have been found to be effective in the laboratory and in clinical trials in moderately severe asthma.[79] A number of agents are under investigation. Two agents have been included in the latest NHLBI guidelines as alternative first line anti-inflammatory treatments for long term control and prevention of symptoms in mild persistent asthma in adults and in children over 12 years of age. These are zafirlukast, a leukotriene receptor antagonist which acts as a selective competitive inhibitor of LTD4 and LTE4 receptors, and zilueton which is a 5-lipoxygenase inhibitor. These recommendations increase the possible range of anti-inflammatory treatments in mild asthma but further work on comparisons with inhaled steroids is needed.

Liver enzymes should be monitored on zilueton therapy and it can inhibit metabolism of terfenadine, warfarin and theophylline. Zafirlukast should be taken at least one hour before or two hours after meals as food decreases the bioavailability.

Oral anti-allergics

Antihistamines may act as antimediator drugs. An important example is ketotifen, which is an oral nonselective antihistamine that may have a more broad anti-allergic mechanism. Pharmacologically it has actions similar to sodium cromoglycate and nedocromil and thus it can be classed as anti-inflammatory. Whatever the merits of this argument, clinically it only has, at best, minor effectiveness compared with placebo. Its use in children may reflect its benefits in treating eczema and rhinitis. Many other oral anti-allergic treatments are available, especially in Japan. In the absence of randomized placebo comparison with existing inhaled anti-inflammatory medication the role of this treatment must remain uncertain.

Alpha blockers

Alpha receptors are present in the airways, although their extent is small and much debated. Alpha blockers have been tried both by the systemic and inhaled route but to date no useful clinical benefit has been found[80] and therefore this potentially promising line of treatment appears to be ineffective.

Calcium-channel blockers

In recent years there has also been interest in calcium-channel blocking agents. This has arisen because of the realization that mediator release is in part a calcium-dependent mechanism, and interest has been further stimulated by observations that drugs like nifedipine and verapamil can influence bronchial reactivity. These agents have been shown to modify exercise-induced asthma as well as other tests of reactivity.[44,45] They do not appear to alter resting bronchomotor tone and therefore do not act as bronchodilators.

Whether they are effective in clinical practice remains to be determined, although initial clinical experience is not favourable. They do, however, provide a rational approach to the treatment of conditions such as angina and hypertension in patients with asthma, as beta blockers are contraindicated.

Others

Treatment for severe chronic steroid-dependent asthma is unsatisfactory. Various agents have been tried.

- methotrexate
- cyclosporin B
- gold

All have shown some benefit but there is a fear that their long-term side-effects may be added to those of corticosteroids, so the net benefit may be small. Their use remains experimental.

Combined preparations

Oral   For many years a large number of oral combined preparations were available for the treatment of asthma. Many of these contained small doses of ephedrine and theophylline, sometimes together with a subtherapeutic dose of a sedative. These doses are unlikely to achieve satisfactory bronchodilatation. Nevertheless some patients were attached to such treatments, which they may have taken for many years. They are not likely to be harmful unless they delay the use of more appropriate therapy, but there can be no rationale for starting new asthmatic patients on such treatment. Few combined preparations remain on the market.

Inhaled   New combined inhalers are now being produced and are often popular. In general it is undesirable to have asthmatics on combined preparations because asthma is a variable condition in which treatments need to be adjusted to the current state of the disease. These combined preparations may also confuse the patient if they combine preventive and relieving medication. The main arguments in their favour are convenience and an increased use of preventive treatment. Many patients require both an inhaled anti-inflammatory and a bronchodilator, and so combining them, particularly with twice daily medications, is convenient and may aid compliance. This is particularly important for regular inhaled anti-inflammatory treatment whose consumption may be sustained if given with an inhaled bronchodilator.

Bronchial lavage

The contribution of inflammation to asthma with mucus plugging has led to the idea that asthma can be helped by washing out the airways. These lavage procedures are also sometimes carried out in the rare patient who may require ventilation. Interest in this approach has been sustained by the occasional apparent success and this has led some clinicians to try bronchial lavage in less acutely ill patients, particularly those who may be requiring systemic steroids, in the hope that this step can be avoided. Apart from the occasional favourable report, the bulk of the evidence suggests that this treatment is not successful and may be potentially harmful. The role of washing out mucus plugs remains to be determined and the best procedure for this has not been established (see Chapter 10).

Mucolytic agents

There is no evidence that mucolytic agents provide any beneficial effects in the treatment of either acute or chronic asthma.[81]

Combined inhaled asthma preparations

Aerocrom	salbutamol 100 mcg, sodium cromoglycate 1 mg
Combivent	salbutamol 100 mcg, ipratropium 20 mcg
Duovent + autohaler	fenoterol 100 mcg, ipratropium 40 mcg
Duovent + unit dose vials for nebulizer	fenoterol 1.25 mg, ipratropium 500 mcg per 4 ml
Intal Compound	sodium cromoglycate 20 mg, isoprenaline sulphate 0.1 mg
Ventide + autohaler	beclomethasone diproprionate 50 mcg, salbutamol 100 mcg
Ventide Rotacaps	beclomethasone dipropionate 200 mcg, salbutamol 400 mcg
Ventide Paediatric Rotacaps	beclomethasone dipropionate 100 mcg, salbutamol 200 mcg

PRACTICAL POINTS

- Despite the large number of treatments available for chronic asthma there is still considerable uncertainty about the best approach.
- Important strategic considerations include the need to treat the underlying pathogenesis of asthma, as well as to use inhaled therapy wherever possible to maximize the safety margin of treatment.
- Inhaled treatment with bronchodilators and anti-inflammatory medication, used singly or in combination, will control the vast majority of asthmatic patients. This can provide potent and safe treatment and is far superior to nonpharmacological measures to control asthma.
- Guidelines will assist in the choice of appropriate treatment. These guidelines identify criteria for control of asthma and provide a stepwise therapeutic regimen based on severity.
- Control of chronic asthma requires treatment of its cause. Inhaled anti-inflammatory medication is currently recommended for this purpose.
- The avoidance of risk factors underpins asthma medication and should be advised if appropriate.
- Therapy requires patient education and a policy of self-management. Guidelines and consensus reports provide valuable advice.
- Newer anti-inflammatory agents may be shown to provide an alternative to steroids in mild persistent asthma.

6
Childhood asthma

BACKGROUND

The management of a child with asthma differs from that of an adult in terms of treatment; in addition there are special problems which we shall be reviewing in this chapter. Children are surprisingly tolerant of almost adult doses of drugs but their type of asthma and prognosis is somewhat different. It is also necessary to take into account that children suffering from a chronic disease will have their own emotional and school problems. The main practical problem with childhood asthma, though, appears to be that of diagnosis, or more specifically labelling, and we turn to this first of all.

DIAGNOSIS

Asthma is difficult to diagnose in children below twelve months of age. Under this age infants often wheeze with upper respiratory infections because their small airways are easily obstructed by a little mucus or oedema of the bronchial wall. Most such children do not respond well to beta$_2$ agonists. Over one-third suffer from asthma later in childhood. Above the age of twelve months recurrent bouts of wheezing should always be regarded as asthma unless there is good evidence to contradict this.

Several studies have indicated a reluctance to make the diagnosis of asthma in children.[18,19] This stems from a false complacency about the benign nature of wheezing in children and a feeling that the diagnostic label of 'asthma' causes anxiety to the parents. Consequently the term 'wheezy bronchitis' is often used instead and appropriate asthmatic treatment withheld.

There have been a number of studies demonstrating that children with asthma may present solely with cough, particularly during the night,[7] and therefore any child who has repeated attacks of coughing and in whom the diagnosis of recurrent bronchitis is made should be suspected of having asthma.

The importance of recognizing cough as a presenting symptom of asthma in childhood should not however obscure the fact that the classic asthmatic symptoms of wheezing and dyspnoea are not that uncommon in children. In two surveys of schoolchildren aged between seven and nine years 11 per cent were found to have episodes of wheezing, but surprisingly few of these children had been labelled as asthmatic.[18] It is essential to consider the diagnosis of asthma in any child who has a persistent cough or episodes of

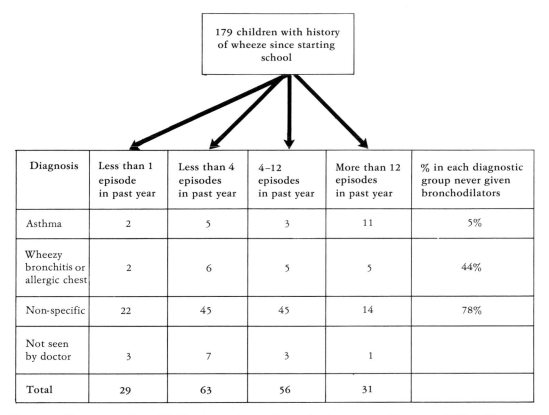

Diagnosis	Less than 1 episode in past year	Less than 4 episodes in past year	4–12 episodes in past year	More than 12 episodes in past year	% in each diagnostic group never given bronchodilators
Asthma	2	5	3	11	5%
Wheezy bronchitis or allergic chest	2	6	5	5	44%
Non-specific	22	45	45	14	78%
Not seen by doctor	3	7	3	1	
Total	29	63	56	31	

Figure 6.1 Doctors are often disinclined to make the diagnosis of asthma, as this series of 179 children demonstrates. The failure to attach the diagnosis of asthma was associated with a failure to prescribe appropriate treatment.

bronchitis associated with wheeze and breathlessness, particularly if these symptoms are disturbing sleep of both child and parents. One or two such episodes may not be sufficient to make the diagnosis of asthma but more attacks than this certainly suggests such a diagnosis and it is then necessary to consider appropriate treatment (Fig. 6.1).

When children with wheezing attacks are correctly labelled as asthmatic and given appropriate treatment their school record improves, family tensions and anxieties are greatly reduced, and the children are more able to lead a normal life.

Fear of labelling

The main problem in childhood asthma is often more one of labelling than diagnosis, as most parents and practitioners probably recognize that a child with recurrent bronchitis may have asthma, but there is a general reluctance to make this diagnosis.

As we have said, this is often based on the fear that this label may have an adverse effect on the child and family, but all the evidence suggests that the correct labelling is of benefit to all concerned. This is because effective treatment is now readily available

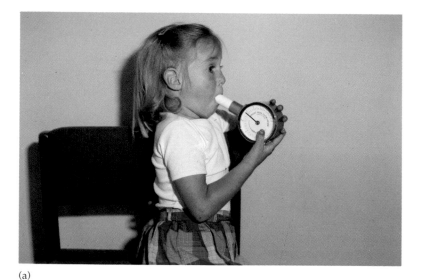

(a)

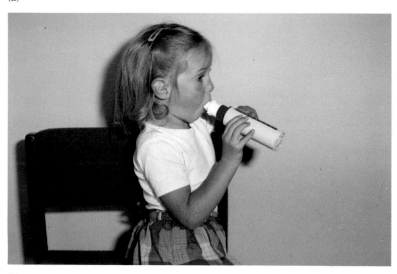

(b)

Figure 6.2 (a) A low-range peak flow meter is available for measuring peak flow rate in children. (b) A portable low-range mini peak flow meter can be used for children or those whose peak flow is consistently low.

which can not only improve symptoms but also minimize the distress caused to the family by those symptoms. The child is able to lead a normal life, play games and go to school. Although this is achieved by the use of drug regimens, these are now extremely safe and easy to administer, and good control of symptoms is clearly preferable to having an untreated invalid child, with all the resulting family worries and the potential loss of lung function and growth retardation caused by poorly controlled asthma.

Special tests

The diagnosis of asthma in childhood, as in adults, can usually be made on the history, but often there are few signs when the child is seen, and then it is useful to search for other diagnostic clues.

Skin tests   Most children with asthma are atopic and therefore skin testing might help, as negative results can suggest an alternative diagnosis (see Chapter 8).

Peak flow   Measurement of peak flow can be useful, particularly if taken by the parent during an attack, so that the variability of lung function is clearly seen (Fig. 6.2). If the peak flow is lower than predicted, a response to inhaled bronchodilator can be assessed which may also demonstrate lung function variability.

Airway challenge   Sometimes it may also be helpful to challenge the airways. Most children will demonstrate exercise-induced asthma if appropriately tested. All that this usually requires is that they run for about five minutes at a sufficient rate to make them breathless and raise their heart rate. If the peak flow is measured before and after exercise, a fall of greater than 15 per cent will be observed some five or ten minutes after stopping exercise if the patient has asthma. This test is particularly useful in those children who have an unexpected intolerance of exercise during school games, as some of them are genuinely unable to compete because of their asthma.

   Only very rarely will more specific challenge be necessary and this is best carried out in specialized units.

Trial of treatment   In the vast majority of children the diagnosis can be satisfactorily made from history and peak flow measurements alone. If there is any doubt it is usually best to carry out a trial of treatment rather than further tests, as a trial is itself often diagnostic. In a child with recurrent episodes of bronchitis the treatment may have to be taken regularly for a number of months to establish its worth but there is usually little doubt in the minds of parent and child if it is successful.

Diagnostic tests for childhood asthma

- Skin tests
- Peak flow monitoring
- Trial of inhaled bronchodilator or sodium cromoglycate
- Airway challenge (e.g. exercise)

ASTHMA TRIGGERS

As with adults, asthma in children may be triggered by a number of factors. Exercise is more frequently an identifiable cause of asthma in children than in adults, as youngsters are more likely to sustain longer periods of muscular exertion; some children therefore present with exercise-induced asthma. The pathogenesis of exercise-induced asthma involves drying and cooling of the airways and therefore it is not surprising that going to school or out to play in the cold winter air may also act as a trigger in some children.

Infections Respiratory infections commonly trigger attacks of asthma and this contributes to the erroneous diagnosis of wheezy bronchitis and consequent unnecessary treatment with antibiotics. These infections are often viral and in many patients a refractory trigger is the only important cause for an exacerbation.

Atopy Many children with asthma are atopic and therefore have associated hay fever and pollen asthma. They are also prone to be hypersensitive to the house dust mite and this may be the major trigger factor, as they are surrounded by this allergen when they go to bed. The mite lives not only in the blankets and mattresses, but also in soft toys that they keep close to their faces, making allergen avoidance particularly difficult for children. Most parents find it virtually impossible to keep the toys and bed free of mites (see Chapter 3).

Psychological factors The psychosomatic view of asthma is felt by some authorities to be particularly important in children. As with adults, emotional distress is not itself a cause of asthma but in an asthmatic individual it may play a role in triggering attacks. Undoubtedly some children use their asthma for secondary gain but these are manipulative children who would use whatever illness or disability was to hand to influence parents and teachers. This type of behaviour is not exclusively associated with asthma.

In general the best way of tackling the emotional disturbance surrounding asthma is to treat asthma effectively, and not to concentrate too much attention on the psychological aspects.

Asthma trigger factors in childhood

- Exercise
- House dust mite
- Pollens
- Respiratory infections
- Animals
- Psychological factors

ASSESSMENT

The assessment of childhood asthma is similar to that of adults and is largely based on the methods used for achieving a diagnosis. Thus a clinical history is very useful in assessing childhood asthma, not only because it helps make the diagnosis but because it can also provide an assessment of severity. The more often the child has attacks of asthma and the greater the accompanying wheeze and dyspnoea, the more severe is the attack (Fig. 6.3). Other important indicators of severity are the amount of sleep disturbance associated with each asthmatic attack, and bronchodilator consumption, which needs to be monitored carefully by the physician.

Date this card was started:	*1 MAY '84*		1	2	3	4	5	6	7
1. WHEEZE LAST NIGHT	Good night .... 0 Slept well but slightly wheezy .... 1 Woke × 2–3 because of wheeze........ 2 Bad night, awake most of time 3		0	0	1	0	0	1	2
2. COUGH LAST NIGHT	None........................... 0 Little .... 1 Moderately bad...................... 2 Severe 3		0	0	0	0	1	2	1
3. WHEEZE TODAY	None........................... 0 Little .... 1 Moderately bad...................... 2 Severe 3		1	0	1	1	0	1	2
4. ACTIVITY TODAY	Quite normal....................... 0 Can only run short distance .... 1 Limited to walking because of chest ... 2 Too breathless to walk............... 3		0	0	0	0	0	1	1
5. NASAL SYMPTOMS	None........................... 0 Mild .... 1 Moderate .... 2 Severe 3		0	0	0	0	1	1	2
6. METER Best of 3 blows	Before breakfast medicines .... Before bedtime medicines		350 400	355 390	360 395	370 410	360 385	340 375	325 335
7. DRUGS Number of doses actually taken during the past 24 hours.	Name of drug Dose prescribed SALBUTAMOL INHALER as necessary PREDNISOLONE 30 mg		4	4	6	6	8	8	12
8. COMMENTS Note if you see a doctor (D) or stay away from school (S) or work (W) because of your chest and anything else important such as an infection (I).									COLD

Figure 6.3 A detailed diary card like this provides a useful record to help monitor the severity of a child's asthma, in this case indicating the need for the addition of anti-inflammatory treatment.

ROUTES OF ADMINISTRATION

In the earlier chapters we have stressed that the best route of administration for asthma therapy is the inhaled route as this minimizes the dose of drug delivered and provides effective treatment with the widest safety margin. We have also emphasized that the vast majority of patients can be treated satisfactorily by the inhaled route using the appropriate medications, either singly or in combination. These principles also apply to the management of childhood asthma, but a number of points specific to children need to be borne in mind.

Difficulties with inhalers

As might be expected, children find inhalers more difficult to use the younger they are. There is no evidence that children aged eight and above are more or less successful than adults with hand-held inhalers, but below that age there are increasing difficulties, and most doctors find it impossible to have children use inhalers if they are younger than three years of age. This applies particularly to pressurized aerosols. Breath-actuated metered dose inhalers may be useful in children.

Other delivery systems suitable for young children

Dry-powder aerosols   Partly because of these difficulties, delivery systems have been introduced that may be of particular help to children with asthma. Dry-powder delivery systems such as the Spinhaler for delivering sodium cromoglycate are actuated by the child's inspiration and therefore more successful in young children. Using a similar principle, the Rotahaler or Diskhaler allow administration of salbutamol and beclomethasone dipropionate. The Turbohaler is an effective multi-dose powder inhaler for terbutaline and budesonide; the Accuhaler can be used for salmeterol and fluticasone. Other powder delivery systems are under development so the majority of children should be able to choose one to enable effective inhaled therapy to be used. In this way children with asthma can obtain the full range of therapy also available to adults. These powdered aerosols have led to a major improvement in the prospects of successful asthma treatment for children below the age of seven years, as they can be used successfully by children down to the age of two to three years.[82]

Nebulizers   There are a number of reservations about the use of nebulizers in the treatment of asthma, but in children this delivery system appears to be particularly successful, especially when asthma is severe. The treatment of severe asthma has therefore been improved by a better understanding of nebulizers and the availability of a full range of treatment.

Spacers   The expense and complexity of nebulizers as well as problems with pressurized aerosols, have also led to the introduction of extension tubes or 'spacers' to be attached to pressurized aerosols. They improve the prospects of inhaling appropriate respirable particles as well as aiding patient compliance and may have a useful part to play if they can supplant the more expensive and complicated nebulizer. The most recent introduction is the Babyhaler, which is designed for infants and small children. As we have mentioned in the previous chapters, there are many new advances being made in delivery system design and we shall be discussing these more fully in Chapter 9.

Environmental control

In children the avoidance of provoking factors is especially important. Not only might it reduce the risk of asthma induction but it might also reduce the need for medication.

The domestic mite is a clearly identifiable risk factor and every effort should be made to reduce exposure. Unfortunately the long-term benefits of mite elimination techniques (such as use of impermeable bedding or removal of carpets and curtains) are not well established. Changes to indoor environment by better ventilation and air dehumidification are also under investigation.

Some risk factors are easily avoided, e.g. the family cat, but often the children and parents prefer treatment of the child to removal of the cause.

TREATMENT

The treatment of childhood asthma is largely based on pharmacological measures and is very similar to that of adults (see Chapter 4 and 5). The improved delivery systems and newer drugs introduced over the last decade or so have radically altered the prospects for asthma therapy so that today very few children are significantly disabled by this condition.

Acute asthma

The management of acute asthma in children involves a greater use of nebulizers and less use of intravenous therapy than in adults. Ipratropium bromide is generally more useful in adults than children but seems to be particularly beneficial in children under eighteen months, when beta$_2$ agonists are less effective.

As with adults, in addition to bronchodilators the prompt administration of an adequate dose of corticosteroid is essential in treating the acute attack and in preventing the deteriorating attack of asthma.

It is very unusual for a child to require ventilator therapy and this is usually best avoided if adequate treatment is given early enough. The same principle applies to the admission of children with asthma to hospital, which should be less frequent with the introduction of effective inhaled treatment.

The main problem for the physician remains one of diagnosis, as effective treatment can only be given once the correct label has been given.

Chronic asthma

Explanation   When children suffer from chronic asthma, drug therapy has to be supplemented by special attention to the child and family. It is therefore particularly important to give as full an explanation as possible to the parents so that they can adequately monitor and supervise therapy. This information also needs to be transmitted to the school authorities to ensure that there is the minimum disruption to school life possible.

To avoid enhancing parents' fears and prejudices concerning asthma, the practitioner should stress that with the effective treatment now available, most children can lead a

MANAGEMENT OF CHRONIC ASTHMA IN CHILDREN UNDER 5 YEARS OF AGE

- Avoidance of provoking factors where possible
- Working towards a self-management plan
- Selection of best inhaler device

Step 1:

Occasional use of relief bronchodilators

Short-acting β agonists 'as required' for symptom relief but not more than once daily. Before altering a treatment step ensure that the patient is taking the treatment, the inhaler is appropriate, and inhaler technique is good. Address any concerns or fears. Mildest cases may respond to oral β agonists.

Step 2:

Regular inhaled preventer therapy

Inhaled short acting β agonists as required
plus:
(i) cromoglycate as powder (20 mg 3–4 times daily) or via metered dose inhaler and large volume spacer (10 mg thrice daily),
or:
(ii) beclomethasone or budesonide up to 400 µg or fluticasone up to 200 µg daily. Consider a 5-day course of soluble prednisolone (dose given above) or temporary increase in inhaled steroids (double dose) to gain rapid control.

Step 3:

Increased dose inhaled steroids

Inhaled short-acting β agonists as required
plus:
beclomethasone or budesonide increased to 800 µg or fluticasone 500 µg daily via a large volume spacer. Consider short prednisolone course. Consider adding regular twice daily long acting β agonist or a slow release xanthine.

Figure 6.4 British Thoracic Society Guidelines on the management of chronic asthma in children. (Reproduced with permission from ref. 57.)

Starting out:
Patients should start treatment at the step most appropriate to the initial severity. A rescue course of prednisolone may be needed at any step (<1 year 1–2 mg/kg/day; 1–5 years 20 mg/day).

Step 4:

High-dose inhaled steroids and bronchodilators

Inhaled steroids (up to 2 mg/day) and other treatment as in step 3. Slow release xanthines or nebulised β agonists.

Stepping down

Regularly review the need to decrease treatment and step down as indicated. Monitor all changes in treatment by clinical review.

normal life. He should also involve the parents in decisions on management and make sure that they know precisely what to do when control of asthma deteriorates. Patient education and self-management in the context of the family is particularly important.

Medication   To achieve adequate control of asthma attacks, the child must learn how to use an inhaler correctly. As mentioned above, in the younger child this is more likely to happen if the child is prescribed a powder inhaler, but whichever inhaler is used the child must know how to use it satisfactorily. Once the technique has been mastered the child can use his inhaler not only to treat acute episodes with a selective beta$_2$ agonist such as salbutamol, but also to take the appropriate suppressive inhaled drugs on a regular basis.

As with adult asthma, guidelines for the management of childhood asthma have been drawn up (Fig. 6.4). These have been taken from the revised British Thoracic Society Guidelines published in 1997.[57] The main difference from the adult guidelines is in the use of inhaled steroids, which are used more cautiously in children.

Effects of corticosteroids on childhood growth   The main reservations about prescribing corticosteroids in childhood asthma are that growth may be affected, and that children may experience the other systemic side-effects seen in adults.

The introduction of inhaled beclomethasone dipropionate in 1972 has probably changed the balance of the benefits and side-effects of corticosteroid treatment, especially as far as stunting of growth is concerned. During the first decade of use of beclomethasone dipropionate, a number of studies were carried out and no convincing interference with growth was established following regular administration of inhaled steroids. Growth is in fact promoted in some patients as asthma is brought under control because of the well-known effect of asthma itself stunting growth.[83]

Oral corticosteroids, on the other hand, undoubtedly can stunt growth, even when given on alternate days to minimize side-effects.

The use of higher doses of inhaled steroids and further studies looking at asthma management and the effect on growth have led to inhaled steroids being used more cautiously. While sodium cromoglycate is still extensively used as preventive anti-inflammatory therapy, on balance, inhaled steroids are more effective and will restore health and lung function more frequently than sodium cromoglycate. A recent 8-week study with fluticasone propionate has established its greater efficacy over sodium cromoglycate without the recruitment of side-effects.[73] However, clinical trials over years are required to establish the respective roles of each anti-inflammatory treatment.

Sedation   In adults with asthma, sedation is contraindicated as it is largely without value and is potentially dangerous. The same considerations apply to children with asthma, although sedatives do appear to have some success in controlling symptoms, which may account for the widespread use of antihistamine-containing cough mixtures. As a treatment for asthma, sedation is not particularly effective and certainly much less so than asthma medication. In view of the potential hazard from sedation, agents such as antihistamines should not be given, because more effective anti-asthmatic therapy is available without this particular side-effect.

Antibiotic treatment

The susceptibility of children to respiratory tract infections is well known, as is the association of asthma with some of these infections. This observation coupled with the diagnosis often made of wheezy bronchitis usually leads to antibiotics being prescribed. The failure of this treatment to alter the natural history of the wheezing episode should lead to the correct diagnosis of asthma but also indicates the unfortunate fact that antibiotics are of no value in managing asthmatic attacks produced by viral infections. Antibiotics should therefore only be used for a suspected bacterial infection rather than the asthma attack produced by it. In other words, when antibiotics are required on the basis of the infection they should be given, but they should not be given solely for the treatment of asthma, as there is little evidence that antibiotics play a useful role in these circumstances.

What to do

- The value of drug treatment is greatly enhanced if adequate time and care are given in educating the child and parents about the need for treatment and how it can best be used.
- Patient education should also embrace a better understanding of asthma itself and how it can be avoided, but unfortunately environmental control is seldom of great success.
- The treatment of childhood asthma is very similar to that for adults. Inhaled bronchodilators for attacks or in combination with inhaled anti-inflammatory treatment for chronic asthma can control the majority of children very successfully and with little risk of side-effects.
- Oral theophylline therapy may be more effective in children than in adults but the dose needs to be carefully monitored to avoid toxic side-effects.
- Low-dose inhaled steroids appear to have little effect on growth but this issue is not entirely resolved.
- Sedation is not a potent form of asthma treatment and is potentially harmful, so it is best avoided.
- Desensitization is also unlikely to be of help (see Chapter 8).

PROGNOSIS

About 50 per cent of children with asthma grow out of it and most of the rest find that its force lessens once puberty has passed. The excess of boys with asthma in childhood is lost by adulthood, indicating that improvement in asthma is particularly likely to occur in males.

Unfortunately, in a significant proportion, asthma returns in later life. The condition recurs in a third of asthmatics who have at least a year completely free of symptoms. Patients should be aware of this to prevent their adult asthma from being underdiagnosed and therefore undertreated.

PRACTICAL POINTS

- Childhood asthma is underdiagnosed and undertreated.
- A cough may be the only presenting symptom in childhood asthma.
- Over the age of seven years most children can manage to use a metered dose inhaler. Many younger children can also be taught the technique.
- Alternative devices such as dry powder systems allow many children as young as two to three years of age to use inhaled treatment.
- Nebulizers are useful at any age.
- Most children with asthma are atopic and attention should be paid to identifying and avoiding allergens which are found to precipitate their asthma.
- Around half of all children with asthma grow out of it.
- Asthma treatment guidelines for children are similar to those for adults, but recommend greater caution concerning use of inhaled steroids.
- Education of child and parents is the key to success.

7
Asthma in general practice

Most of the management of asthma is carried out by general practitioners. With the high prevalence of asthma the workload dictates that hospital chest clinics cannot deal with most patients. In most cases, good asthma control can be established on regular inhaled therapy and therefore hospital attendance is unnecessary. General practitioners have a particularly important role in making the initial diagnosis of asthma and are in the best position to deal with the general management of asthmatic patients. Hospital specialists should work in collaboration with their local general practitioners and take on the more severe cases or those with particular problems.

Some studies in the early 1980s suggested that care in general practice could be improved. The British Thoracic Association study of asthma deaths found that severity of symptoms prior to death was not always appreciated by general practitioners.[24] Other work showed a reluctance to use the term asthma associated with inadequate prescription of appropriate asthma therapy. The advent of clinical audit in hospitals showed that these deficiencies in asthma care were certainly not restricted to general practitioners. Over the last ten years this reluctance to use the label asthma has decreased. Guidelines have been published for the management of childhood and adult asthma[57] and the general feeling is that asthma care has improved as a result of these and other developments. Many general practitioners have set up asthma clinics run by trained nurses or interested doctors where asthma care can be developed and more time spent with individual patients.

ASTHMA CLINICS

In the UK the government encouraged the development of specialized clinics in general practice covering common conditions such as asthma. Most of these asthma clinics are run by a practice nurse. Often one partner in a group practice develops a particular interest in asthma and supervises the clinic. Training for nurses can be arranged at local chest clinics, and the Stratford-upon-Avon Asthma Training Centre (see page 156) has developed very successful courses which many practice nurses have attended.

A group practice of 10,000 patients would expect to have up to 500 recognized asthmatic patients. If half of these came just twice a year this would provide a busy weekly asthma clinic. Asthmatics should be identified at surgery visits, from hospital letters and from prescribing databases. Clinics will need to be arranged at convenient times since many patients will be at work or at school. Protocols for practice nurses should be developed. These should include the development and supervision of management plans, and the checking of home peak flow recordings, diary cards and inhaler technique. Nurses running asthma clinics will need to have ready access to advice from their general practitioners and guidelines for the limits of the nurses' role should be established. This will vary between practices and will depend on such aspects as the training the nurse has received.

It is often helpful for the nurse to have contact with the local chest clinic staff. Many hospital clinics now have their own community liaison nurses who deal with severe cases at home and will need to communicate with practice asthma clinics.

A large part of the care in an asthma clinic will involve education and encouragement of the patient in their treatment. Self-management plans can be developed for each patient, giving indications for adjustments to treatment or for consultation with doctor or nurse, based on symptoms and objective peak flow criteria. Attempts have been made to demonstrate the benefit of the supervision and care delivered by asthma clinics. This is not an easy task since adequate control data is not usually available. However, there is increasing evidence that supervision and management plans do improve care when they concentrate on practical aspects. Earlier work showed that provision of information about the underlying pathology and pharmacology of asthma improved patients' knowledge without necessarily improving asthma management or compliance with treatment. A more practical approach directed at individual patient's needs is likely to be more useful.

It is sensible to audit the work of a practice asthma clinic. This audit can look at the coverage of the patients with asthma within a practice and at the adherence to locally or nationally established management guidelines within the clinic. More elaborate studies of clinic effectiveness require larger collaborative work.

WHO SHOULD BE REFERRED TO HOSPITAL?

This is one area where it can be helpful to set up local guidelines with the nearby chest physicians and paediatricians. Readiness to refer appropriately will depend on the organization of the local chest clinic as well as the practice. There is little to be gained from a series of hospital visits to see a succession of senior house officers rather than visits to a general practitioner who knows the history and the home circumstances in detail.

Referral for diagnostic problems

When there are doubts about the underlying diagnosis, referral can be useful. Simple exercise tests can be carried out in practice, but more complicated lung function testing usually requires access to a respiratory function laboratory. In some cases, challenge testing with methacholine or histamine may be appropriate. When alternative diagnoses such as cystic fibrosis are being considered a referral is appropriate.

When there is suspicion that an occupational element is involved then an experienced chest physician should usually be involved.

In older patients with wheezing where there are doubts about the diagnosis, referral for lung function testing, diagnostic imaging or even bronchoscopy may be appropriate. This should be the case if there is any suspicion of obstruction of a large airway.

Referral based on severity

The level of severity at which referral to hospital is appropriate depends on the expertise and experience of the general practitioner and arrangements made with local chest physicians. In general, referral should occur for those patients who need oral steroid courses more than two or three times a year, those who require inhaled steroid doses above 800 mcg beclomethasone dipropionate daily (or equivalent), and those for whom home nebulizer use or chronic oral steroid therapy is being considered.

Patients whose asthma has been severe enough to be admitted to hospital should generally be seen in a hospital chest clinic after discharge. There is evidence that involvement of a trained respiratory physician rather than a general physician in hospital and outpatient care improves the control and readmission rate in such patients.

Other problems

Pregnant patients with deteriorating asthma, patients with brittle asthma who have severe, sudden attacks and those whose asthma interferes with their life style despite treatment should usually be referred to hospital.

PRACTICE EQUIPMENT FOR ASTHMA MANAGEMENT

The use of nebulizers at home is contentious. They can be used for delivery of bronchodilators in acute exacerbations or for regular therapy. Any asthmatic with their own nebulizer at home must understand exactly when it should be used and in what circumstances further help is needed. The worry is that a patient will stay at home using their nebulizer when other treatment is necessary. When a home nebulizer is being considered, hospital referral is usually appropriate and facilities for maintenance of the machine need to be organized.

Most practices find it helps to have nebulizers available at the surgery. The practice nurse should have one easily available with a supply of salbutamol and ipratropium bromide nebulizer solutions. They can be used for patients who present with mild to moderate exacerbations but who do not need hospital admission, and for more severe cases to deliver bronchodilators while waiting for transport to hospital. It is useful to have a small supply of nebulizers to lend to patients being treated at home for their exacerbations. This needs to be combined with corticosteroid therapy and careful monitoring of progress. When patients are going away from home to a situation without a reliable electricity supply, an adaptation for a car battery or a footpump-driven nebulizer may be used, although considerable effort is necessary to provide an adequate flow with the footpump.

The cause of death in acute exacerbations of asthma is hypoxia. It is useful to have a small cylinder to provide an emergency supply of oxygen to patients with severe exacerbations while their move to hospital is organized.

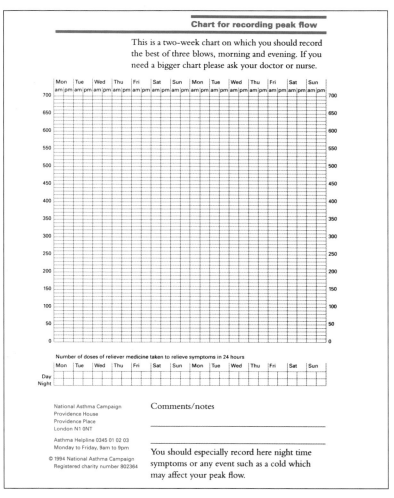

Figure 7.1 Chart for recording peak flow and diary card from the National Asthma Campaign. A simple guide can be entered on an asthma `credit card' for patients to carry at all times.

Peak flow meters for named patients can be obtained on prescription. A general practitioner should have peak flow meters readily available in the surgery and in the asthma clinic. The scales on most commercially available peak flow meters are not calibrated to provide an accurate reading of flow throughout the range. However, one meter provides relatively consistent readings and there is reasonable agreement between the meters from one manufacturer. It is best, therefore, to stick to one make of peak flow meter throughout a practice. Peak flow meters are best used with diary cards to record simple symptom information and drug use with peak flow readings. This allows an assessment of the accuracy of the patient's perception of their own asthma. This is useful in the development of a management plan. Various diary cards are available, such as the one available from the National Asthma Campaign (Fig. 7.1).

It is also useful to have a spirometer available in the practice. This should provide a trace of volume against time or flow against volume. Spirometry is more informative in patients with severe chronic bronchitis and emphysema and the trace can be used to detect occasional patients whose large airway obstruction mimics asthma (see page 5).

The practice nurse will need a variety of placebo inhalers in order to find the appropriate device for each patient. These can be obtained from pharmaceutical companies who are only too happy to encourage the use of their own products.

CONSEQUENCES OF GOOD CARE

The recognition that airway inflammation is an important element in asthma and the consequent increased importance of inhaled steroids in the treatment have led to a change in prescribing habits. In the 1970s and early 1980s prescription of bronchodilators increased markedly. In the late 1980s and the 1990s prescriptions for prophylactic agents increased. There has also been a move away from metered dose inhalers towards dry powder and patient-actuated devices. Both these moves are associated with increased prescribing costs.

General practitioners who have an interest in asthma and those who have started asthma clinics have generally seen an increase in their expenditure on asthma drugs. This is the introduction of appropriate care to a wider group of patients and is quite justified. Practitioners who promote the proper management of asthma in their practices must be prepared for such a rise in prescribing costs. It should be matched by an improvement in asthma control and a reduction in emergency calls and in hospital admissions for exacerbations of asthma which will reduce total costs.

LIAISON WITH HOSPITAL DOCTORS

Many practices have developed close relationships with their local hospital colleagues. This has taken a number of forms. Some chest physicians come out to do joint chest clinics in surgeries and can deal with difficult asthma problems on these visits. Others have worked out joint management protocols and the chest physicians provide easily accessible advice or have regular meetings with their general practice colleagues.

Communication is not always so well established with accident and emergency (A&E) departments. The asthmatics who attend A&E regularly are often those who have not built up a good relationship with their general practitioner or practice nurse and have not worked out a proper management plan. Formal feedback to general practitioners from A&E often goes astray. The situation can be helped by including A&E staff in the development of the local management protocols for asthma.

8
Inflammation and allergy

BACKGROUND

It has been recognized for many years that immunological aspects are important in asthma. Early work produced the chance of therapeutic intervention with sodium cromoglycate which was thought to act by preventing degranulation of mast cells.

The immunological aspects must not be considered in isolation. Asthma can present in many forms and it is possible that there are fundamental differences in aetiology between groups of patients. In all cases, there seems to be a complicated interaction between immunology, reflex nervous changes, underlying differences in bronchial smooth muscle and the development of pathological changes.

CELLULAR INVOLVEMENT

Recognition of the inflammatory aspects of asthma has brought together the cellular, immunological and pathological aspects of asthma. Whereas the response to nonspecific stimuli such as cold air, histamine or methacholine involves only an early response, when the challenge is by inhalation of an allergen such as pollen or house dust mite the early airway narrowing is often followed by a later response. This late asthmatic reaction (LAR) occurs six to nine hours after a single challenge with allergen. It seems to be closer to the situation in spontaneous asthma and is a complicated process involving a number of cell types. The early asthmatic reaction (EAR) occurs within thirty minutes and resolves over the next hour or two. This early response to an allergic stimulus is probably produced through mast cell activation.

Bronchoalveolar lavage and biopsy studies during both remission and induced asthma have provided further evidence on the cellular involvement in asthma. Eosinophils, neutrophils, macrophages, lymphocytes and epithelial cells, as well as mast cells, may all have important roles to play in the coordinated response. The inflammatory change in the airway seems to be the underlying problem that produces the increased reactivity of the asthmatic airway. Products of the cells are also responsible for the damage to the airway wall demonstrated in biopsy and autopsy specimens.

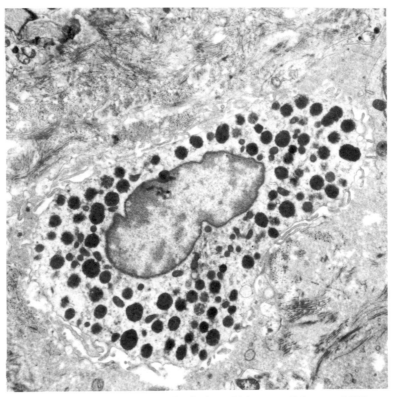

Figure 8.1 An electron micrograph of a bronchial mast cell (mag: x 6,500).

MAST CELLS AND MEDIATORS

Mast cells can be found throughout the bronchial tree and throughout the wall of the airways (Fig. 8.1). They are even found free in the lumen. The granules of the mast cells contain various preformed mediators, and these are released when an appropriate antigen binds to an antibody in order to bridge two adjacent IgE molecules attached to the mast cell surface.

Histamine, neutrophil chemotactic factor and platelet-activating factor released from the granules are all very potent substances capable of producing bronchoconstriction. They are released in sensitized asthmatic subjects on antigen challenge, and in some cases with exercise.[84,85]

Arachidonic acid metabolites

A second group of mediators is produced by mast cell stimulation. These are metabolites of arachidonic acid derived from the cell membrane. Arachidonic acid may be metabolized down either of two pathways (Fig. 8.2). The lipoxygenase pathway leads to

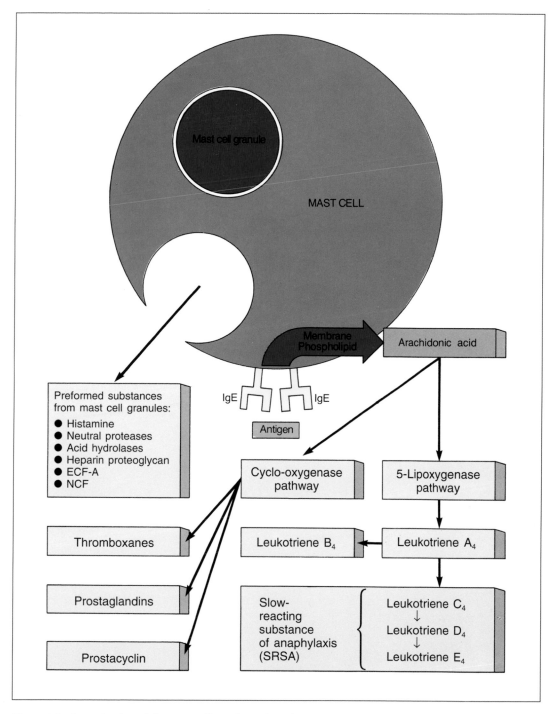

Figure 8.2 On activation of the mast cell, performed mediators are released from granules and new mediators are generated from arachidonic acid.

the production of leukotrienes. These are a group of peptidolipids, the combined activity of which was previously known as a slow-reacting substance of anaphylaxis (SRSA). Several of these leukotrienes can produce bronchoconstriction in very small quantities. Antagonists provide a possible avenue for treatment. Drugs available currently act as inhibitors of 5-lipoxygenase, reducing production of leukotrienes, or as competitive inhibitors of LTE4 and LTD4 receptors.

Metabolism down the cyclo-oxygenase pathway produces prostacyclin, prostaglandins and thromboxane. Different prostaglandins produce either bronchoconstriction or bronchodilatation. The balance between the various pathways of arachidonic acid metabolism is disturbed in the precipitation of asthma by aspirin and related drugs (see Chapter 3).

Eosinophils

Eosinophils are found in increased numbers in the alveolar lavage fluid and the airway wall in asthma. They are in activated form and lose their granules after allergen challenge. This is consistent with discharge of the damaging substances such as major basic protein and eosinophil cationic protein. Interleukin-5 (IL-5) is an important stimulus for the allergic response increasing eosinophil production and recruitment to the lung. Drugs which block IL-5 and IL-4 are being developed for asthma and other inflammatory conditions. Chemokines involved in eosinophil chemotaxis are another target for drug development.

Neutrophils

Neutrophils are attracted to the airway by neutrophil chemotactic factor released from mast and other cells. Neutrophils are recruited into the airways in asthmatic responses but they do not persist and may well be less important than eosinophils.

Macrophages

Alveolar macrophages are activated in asthma and increased numbers are recruited from circulating blood monocytes. The activated macrophages can produce inflammatory mediators, chemotactic factors and cytokines, all of which may be involved in the asthmatic airway response.

Lymphocytes

Present evidence suggests that lymphocytes are important in the orchestration of the inflammatory response rather than being sources of large quantities of inflammatory mediators themselves.

Epithelial cells

Epithelial cells are shed more easily in the inflammatory environment of the asthmatic airway. Epithelial cell loss is a consistent finding in bronchial biopsies in asthma. The epithelium seems to be able to produce endothelin, a vasoconstrictor and bronchoconstrictor, and nitric oxide (NO), a vasodilator and bronchodilator. NO production may be stimulated by locally released cytokines, and the NO produced has cytotoxic effects on the epithelium. NO may also be a transmitter in the nonadrenergic, noncholinergic nervous system.

INTERACTION WITH NERVES

The other important element to be considered in the epithelium is the nervous input. Three types of neural mechanism are involved in control of the airways. The cholinergic fibres constrict smooth muscle. Stimulation of beta adrenoceptors dilates the muscle. There is little or no adrenergic nerve supply to bronchial smooth muscle, so circulating adrenaline provides the main stimulus to these receptors. The third system is the nonadrenergic, noncholinergic (NANC) system, which has various transmitters that can produce constriction or dilatation. It is likely that there is an interaction between the inflammatory aspects of asthma and the neural mechanisms. There may be neurogenic inflammation, and inflammatory mediators may affect the release of neurotransmitters.

IMMUNOLOGICAL TESTS

Skin tests

Immediate skin prick tests are often used in the investigation of asthma. There are two main indications for skin tests:

1. They will confirm the diagnosis of atopy, which itself is a predisposing factor for extrinsic asthma.
2. Positive skin tests may help to confirm a sensitivity suspected from the clinical history.

The mere discovery of a positive skin test by itself does not establish the relevance of that allergen in provoking asthma. A detailed history is much more important. On the other hand, when an inhaled allergen is important it is usual to find a positive skin test. This is not the case for some ingested allergens such as foods, when important sensitivities may exist with negative skin tests.

How they are done   Prick testing is a painless, bloodless procedure (Fig. 8.3). A drop of the extract is placed on the skin and a needle is used to lift up the superficial layers of the epidermis through the drop. It has been estimated that 10^{-6} ml of extract is introduced into the skin. Scratch tests are slightly simpler to perform but more difficult to standardize, so prick tests are generally preferred.

The response is measured as the maximal diameter of the wheal produced in fifteen minutes or the mean of two measurements at right angles. Itching often starts earlier than this, and the whole wheal and flare reaction subsides after one or two hours. Late reactions some hours afterwards occasionally occur.

Immediate skin reactions are produced by specific IgE antibodies releasing mediators from mast cells (see Fig 8.4 for skin prick test results). Atopic subjects usually show positive skin tests to a range of antigens. In Britain, 90 per cent of subjects with any positive tests will be detected by using just four common allergens:[86]

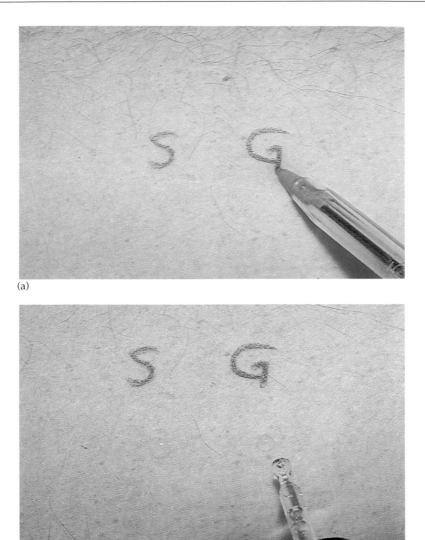

(a)

(b)

Figure 8.3 Skin testing technique.
(a) Careful labelling is essential in the performance of skin prick tests.
(b) A drop of the test solution is placed on the skin.

- Grass pollen
- House dust mite
- *Aspergillus fumigatus*
- Any pet that the subject may be in contact with.

Approximately 20 to 30 per cent of the population will produce at least one skin prick wheal of 3mm diameter. A control solution should always be used to exclude a false

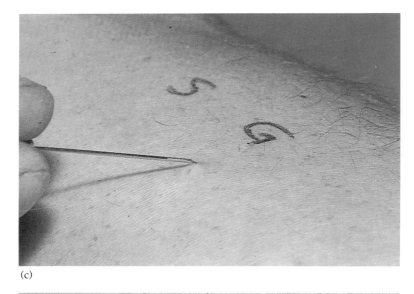

(c)

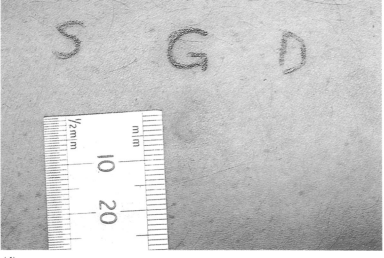

(d)

(c) The superficial layers of the epidermis are raised by the tip of the needle. This is a painless, bloodless procedure.
(d) The diameter of the wheal produced is measured after fifteen minutes.

positive resulting from dermatographia, which is found in about 2 per cent of the population. Size and rate of positive reactions tend to decrease with age.

Of the drugs used in the treatment of asthma, only antihistamines have a significant inhibitory effect on immediate skin tests. They should be discontinued at least twenty-four hours before testing, and this can be confirmed by using a prick test with histamine. In particular, being a Type I hypersensitivity reaction that relies on IgE antibodies, skin prick tests are not affected by corticosteroid treatment.

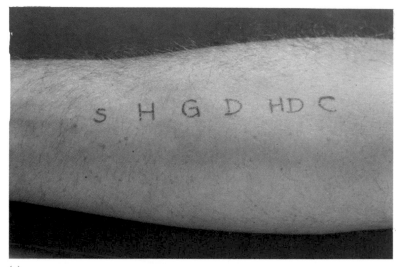

(a)

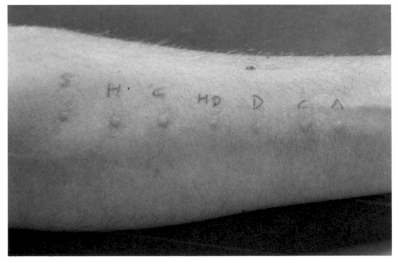

(b)

Figure 8.4 Skin prick test results.
(a) When the histamine control fails to produce a wheal the patient should be questioned about the possible use of antihistamines.
(b) In dermatographia all prick tests, including the saline control, produce similar wheals.

Radioallergosorbent tests (RASTs)

Total IgE levels are raised in 70 per cent of those with extrinsic asthma, and in 5 to 10 per cent of those with intrinsic asthma. The RAST measures the amount of specific IgE to the antigen being investigated. The RAST has a very limited role in the routine management of asthma.[87] It is a relatively expensive test, and in a way is a step back

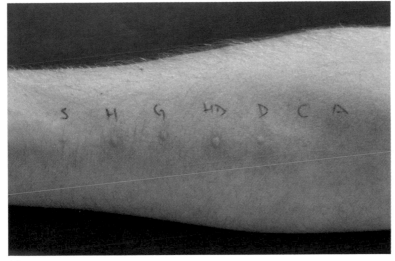

(c)

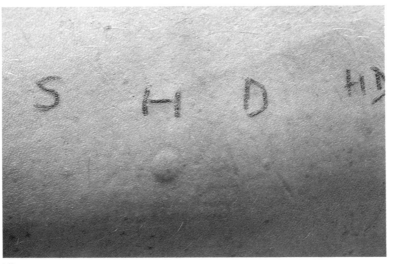

(d)

(c) Most extrinsic asthmatic patients show positive responses to a number of allergens.

(d) A negative skin test response only shows a wheal with the histamine control solution.

from the skin test, which looks at a combination of the IgE level and the ability of this IgE to release active mediators from mast cells in the presence of specific allergen. The RAST measures the specific IgE levels alone (Fig. 8.5).

Most inhaled allergens produce similar results on skin testing and with the RAST. However, in some food sensitivities, the skin test and the RAST may produce conflicting results. The presence of a positive RAST does not establish the importance of an

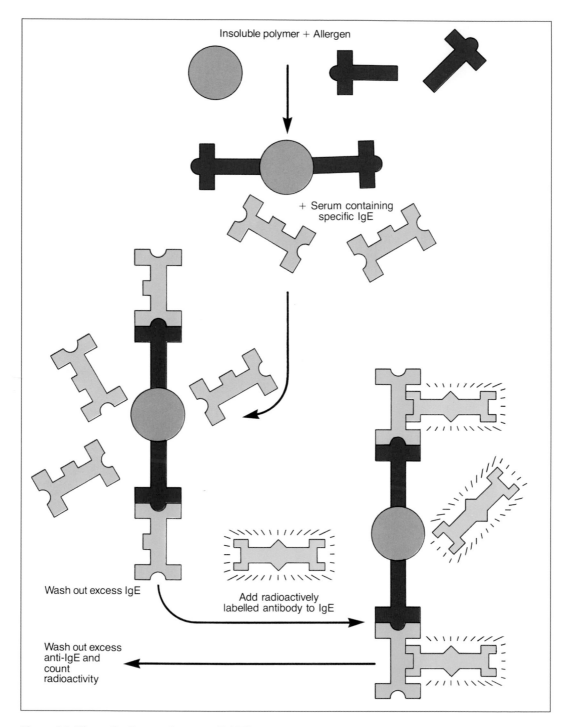

Figure 8.5 The radioallergosorbent test (RAST).

allergen in provoking the patient's asthma. Evidence from the results of exposure or withdrawal are needed for this and, at present, the RAST remains largely a research tool. There is no justification for the preparation of complicated mixtures for hyposensitization on the basis of RAST results.

There are various other radioisotope tests for IgE and IgG but none in widespread use.

Bronchial challenge

Direct evidence of sensitivity of the airways to allergen is provided by bronchial challenge. In this technique small quantities of the suspected allergen are inhaled and respiratory function tests then followed.[88]

Bronchial challenge is not a technique to be undertaken lightly. Firstly, there is the problem of the purification of the antigen and the choice of the initial dose. This may be helped by observing the response to skin testing but unpredictable severe reactions still sometimes occur. The other problem is the occurrence of late reactions about six hours after the challenge. Patients need to be kept under observation over this period after each single challenge exposure.

These problems restrict the use of challenge tests to special experienced laboratories. Allergen challenge is an important research tool in the investigation of the underlying mechanisms of asthma, particularly the inflammatory changes invoked in the late responses. The two clinical situations where they may find a place are in the investigation of occupational asthma (see Chapter 3) and when hyposensitization therapy is being considered.

HYPOSENSITIZATION THERAPY

Background

For over seventy years injection of extracts of sensitizing agents such as pollen has been attempted as a treatment for asthma. It is a much more attractive concept to remove underlying sensitivities in asthma than to suppress the resulting reactions with drugs. Unfortunately many of the claims for the success of hyposensitization are little better than anecdotal reports and few convincing studies exist.[36,37]

The proposed mechanism for hyposensitization is the production of specific IgG antibodies which block the damaging reaction between antigen and IgE antibody. However, attempts to relate improvement to the IgG level, IgE level or some combination of the two have not been convincing.[89] With prolonged treatment IgE levels may decline. An alternative suggestion has been that IgA may be produced. IgA is the antibody found at mucosal surfaces and in secretions. The production of specific IgA might block the penetration of antigen through bronchial or nasal epithelia.

Patient selection   Some of the poor results of hyposensitization may be related to patient selection. Only where one sensitivity is of prime importance in a patient's asthma can hyposensitization hope to work. The majority of asthmatics have many precipitating factors for their wheezing and the removal of one factor makes little difference. In circumstances where a single specific sensitivity is identifiable, such as those people who develop problems after bee and wasp stings, hyposensitization can be very successful. Subjective assessment of response must take account of the large placebo effect produced by a course of regular injections.

How it is done   The usual method of attempting hyposensitization is by the subcutaneous injection of increasing doses of appropriate allergen. Local hyposensitization by way of the nose in rhinitis, or the airways in asthma, has not been successful. On the rare occasions when hyposensitization is successful, the bronchial reactivity to the allergen is reduced. The immunological mechanisms behind changes in reactivity are unclear.

Allergen preparation   One of the many problems with hyposensitization is identification of the allergen to use, and then its purification. Pollen grains and house dust mites contain many potential allergens. When purified the allergens can be chemically modified by formalin, urea or ultraviolet light to produce allergoids. These allergoids have the advantage that, while they continue to induce an immune response, their capacity for producing the allergic reactions is reduced. This can reduce the number of injections required in a course of hyposensitization.

Reactions   Every year there are reports of severe reactions during hyposensitization therapy. Minor local reactions such as pain and swelling at the site of the injection are quite common and call for adjustment of the dosage schedule. Severe anaphylactic reactions are uncommon but may be fatal. In most cases they result from inappropriate use of the preparations, either too high a dose or injection intramuscularly or intravenously. The manufacturer's instructions concerning timing and concentration of injections must be followed carefully. Whenever hyposensitizing injections are given, facilities for resuscitation must be available. Antihistamines may suppress a mild reaction but if an anaphylactic reaction occurs, 0.5–1 ml of 1 in 1,000 adrenaline should be given subcutaneously or intramuscularly and repeated in a few minutes if necessary. Patients should always be observed for one hour after desensitizing injections.

House dust mite desensitization

The house dust mite provides the most common positive skin test in asthma. Although mite levels may vary during the year, the symptoms are perennial and timing of hyposensitization is not likely to be important. Most trials of house dust or house dust mite hyposensitization in adult asthma have shown no benefit.[90] Trials in carefully selected groups of children are a little more impressive.[91] In most cases the selection involved bronchial provocation testing. Although house dust mite hyposensitization may be beneficial in highly selected children with severe asthma, equivalent results can usually be obtained with less trouble and risk by inhaled pharmacological therapy[60] (see Chapter 6).

Desensitization to pollens

The constituents of pollen extracts used for hyposensitization must vary according to the local flora. In the United States ragweed pollen extracts have shown some benefit in allergic rhinitis. There is reasonable agreement that with suitable preparations and selected patients, pollen desensitization in allergic rhinitis decreases symptoms and drug therapy. The effect is increased by repeating the treatment over a number of years.

The results are not so convincing in asthma where there is a disturbing lack of consistency between the effects of bronchial provocation tests and the clinical response.[92]

Desensitization to other allergens

There are no satisfactory placebo-controlled trials to assess the effectiveness of hyposensitization to moulds and animal danders. One small study with cat pelt extract produced decreased skin and bronchial sensitivity in all five patients,[93] but had no assessment of clinical effectiveness. Therefore, problems with animals should be dealt with by avoidance, where appropriate (see page 32), rather than immunotherapy.

Some controlled trials have been done with bacterial vaccines.[94] Since most asthmatic episodes triggered by infection are related to viruses it is not surprising that these were unsuccessful.

There is no place for hyposensitization with food extracts or mixtures concocted from skin tests of IgE measurements.[36,37]

ALLERGIC BRONCHOPULMONARY ASPERGILLOSIS (ABPA)

The fungus *Aspergillus* is very widespread in the environment. It is most prevalent in the autumn and winter months, and is particularly abundant in rotting vegetation and compost heaps. Patients who have a history of ABPA should avoid such exposure. *Aspergillus* is associated with a number of pulmonary diseases, but in asthma the major problem is ABPA.[95] There are occasional reports of fungus balls – aspergillomas – forming in the cavities produced by ABPA,[96] and of invasive aspergillosis (chronic necrotizing aspergillosis) in patients on corticosteroid treatment.[97]

In ABPA there is no invasion of lung tissue by *Aspergillus*, but a sensitivity reaction develops against the fungus in the airway. The fungus grows in mucus plugs, which are often rubbery and sticky and of a characteristic brownish colour at their proximal end (Fig. 8.6). ABPA rarely occurs in individuals without a history of asthma.

Diagnosis

This is made on the combination of asthma, transient lung shadowing on the chest radiograph (Figs. 8.7 and 8.8), eosinophilia in blood and/or sputum, and a positive skin prick test to *Aspergillus fumigatus*, often with a late skin reaction also.[95] Further evidence comes from finding the fungus in sputum plugs. Precipitating antibodies to *Aspergillus* may be found in the blood, but these are more typical of aspergillomas.

Natural history

The immunological reaction to *Aspergillus* in the airways produces bronchial wall damage with eosinophilic consolidation and mononuclear cell infiltration in the surrounding lung tissue. The sticky mucus plugs may cause collapse of areas of the lung.

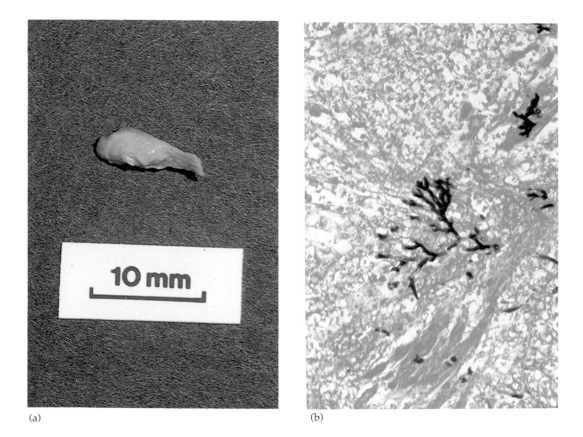

(a)   (b)

Figure 8.6 (a) Firm brownish-coloured plugs are produced in allergic bronchopulmonary aspergillosis (ABPA). (b) Aspergillus can be found growing in the typical ABPA plug.

Continued episodes of ABPA lead to a form of cylindrical bronchiectasis in the affected part of the airway, more proximal than the usual site of bronchiectasis. Prolonged uncontrolled ABPA can lead to lung fibrosis.

Treatment

Acute exacerbations of ABPA can be suppressed by treatment with oral corticosteroids. When episodes are frequent and there is a suggestion of damage producing proximal bronchiectasis, then long-term oral steroid treatment at a dose of 7.5–15 mg daily may be appropriate. An alternative approach may be the use of imidazoles such as itraconazole, since there is some evidence that this may reduce the frequency of episodes of ABPA. Inhaled corticosteroids do not appear to be useful. Patients with infrequent episodes and no evidence of lung damage may not need regular suppressive treatment.

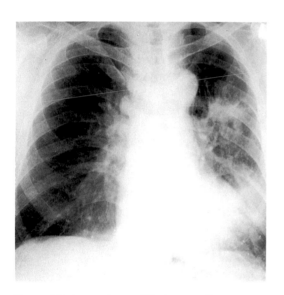

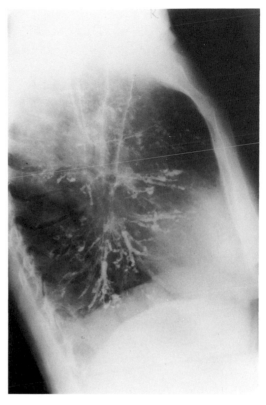

Figure 8.7 Areas of consolidation or collapse may be seen during exacerbations of ABPA.

Figure 8.8 A lateral view of a bronchogram in a patient with ABPA. Recurrent episodes of ABPA have produced bronchiectasis with dilated bronchi showing pooling of contrast medium.

PRACTICAL POINTS

- Airway inflammation plays a key role in asthma pathogenesis.
- The investigation of specific sensitivities relies on the clinical history and skin prick tests in the majority of cases. Occasionally it is necessary to measure IgE levels or assess bronchial reactivity.
- Hyposensitization has, at present, a very limited role to play. It may be useful in house dust mite sensitivity in children and pollen sensitivity, but only in highly selected patients who show response to a single allergen.
- It is to be hoped that further modification of the preparations and understanding of the mechanisms of hyposensitization will lead to better results and a wider application.
- Allergic bronchopulmonary aspergillosis (ABPA) should be considered when there is evidence of pulmonary shadowing with collapse or consolidation in asthma.

9
Methods of drug delivery

BACKGROUND

Many routes of administration can be used for the delivery of drugs in asthma (Fig. 9.1). As with numerous other conditions, it is possible to use oral preparations, suppositories, or injections, either subcutaneous or intravenous. The difference in the treatment of asthma is the availability of the inhaled route, administering the drug directly to its site of action in the lung.

Although most methods of inhalation deliver more drug to the gastrointestinal tract than to the airway, these techniques allow a considerable reduction in the total dose delivered for the same therapeutic effect. This leads to a significant lessening in undesirable systemic side-effects, such as the tremor seen with beta$_2$ agonists. Therefore, as a general rule it is best to use inhaled therapy when possible (Fig. 9.2).

There have been considerable changes in the techniques of delivery of asthmatic therapy, both oral and inhaled, over recent years. For oral therapy this has usually been designed to increase the length of action and tolerance of the preparation. For inhaled therapy most changes have been in the device used for inhalation, trying to increase the delivery to the airways and overcome the problems which some patients have in using this route.

THE GASTROINTESTINAL TRACT

Beta$_2$ agonists

There are considerable disadvantages in using the oral route for beta$_2$ agonists. For an equivalent bronchodilator effect the dose of drug which has to be given is much higher than that used by inhalation.[98] This means that unwanted systemic effects of tremor and tachycardia are much more likely to be troublesome with oral treatment. The other problem is that the onset of action is much slower using tablets[99] and they cannot therefore be used in the same way as inhalers to relieve symptoms quickly.

With the various types of device now available (see subsequent sections), most patients can take their beta$_2$ agonist therapy by inhalation. There remains a place for oral therapy in young children, and where some disability such as failing eyesight or

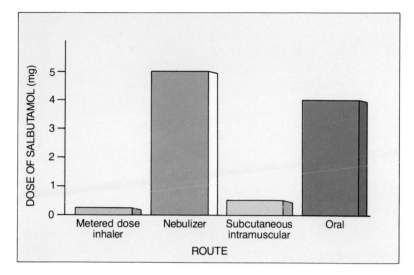

Figure 9.1 Typical single dose of salbutamol given by different routes. This demonstrates the disparity between the dose given by metered dose inhaler and that administered by nebulizer or orally.

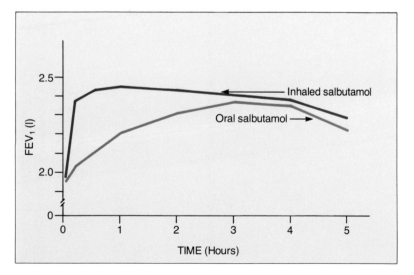

Figure 9.2 Mean change in FEV_1, after oral and inhaled salbutamol in eleven patients.

arthritis makes it difficult to use inhalers. In children, syrups are usually easier to administer than tablets. These should be in the sugar-free form available for salbutamol and terbutaline.

Where nocturnal symptoms are troublesome, it may sometimes be helpful to use slow-release tablets such as salbutamol or agents such as bambuterol with a prolonged action lasting 24 hours, but this is less often necessary with the advent of long-acting inhaled preparations such as salmeterol.

Methylxanthines

Plain theophylline and its ethylenediamine salt, aminophylline, often cause gastro-intestinal upsets when given orally. Some rapid-release preparations such as choline theophyllinate are better tolerated than plain theophylline.

Theophylline and aminophylline suppositories have been used to try to avoid gastric irritation. However, a local irritant proctitis frequently occurs if aminophylline suppositories are used for more than a few days. The absorption of aminophylline from the rectum is erratic and there is no longer any need to use this route now that better tolerated slow-release oral preparations are available.[100]

Many sustained-released preparations of theophylline and aminophylline are now available (see table below). They are associated with fewer side-effects than plain theophylline, although nausea, vomiting and headache may still be a problem. Usually the sustained-release preparations are given on a twelve-hourly regime, or just at night, to stop nocturnal wheezing.[101] However methylxanthines may interfere with the quality of sleep.

Sustained-release preparations of theophylline and aminophylline*

	Tablet size
● **Aminophylline**	
– Pecram	225 mg
– Phyllocontin Continus	225 mg
– Phyllocontin Forte	350 mg
– Phyllocontin Paediatric	100 mg
● **Theophylline**	
– Lasma	300 mg
– Nuelin SA	175 mg, 250 mg
– Slo-Phyllin	60 mg, 125 mg, 250 mg
– Theo-Dur	200 mg, 300 mg
– Uniphyllin Continus	300 mg, 400 mg
– Uniphyllin Paediatric Continus	200 mg

* These formulations vary in the rate and completeness of their absorption; since metabolism also varies between patients drug levels cannot reliably be predicted from the dose given.

The main problems with theophylline therapy are the lack of a sufficient safety margin between the therapeutic range and the toxic range, and the difficulty in predicting the dose necessary to achieve therapeutic levels. There are wide differences in the rate of absorption and the rate of metabolism, and other factors such as smoking and drug therapy may interact (see table below).

Factors affecting theophylline metabolism

- **Increase clearance**
  - Cigarette smoking
  - Marijuana smoking
  - Phenytoin therapy
  - Alcohol

- **Decrease clearance**
  - Erythromycin therapy
  - Cimetidine therapy
  - Ciprofloxacin therapy
  - Allopurinol therapy
  - Frusemide therapy
  - Cirrhosis
  - Cardiac failure
  - Cor pulmonale
  - Sustained fever
  - Old age
  - Neonates
  - Oral contraceptives
  - Influenza vaccine

All patients taking theophylline should have blood levels measured aiming for levels between 8 and 20 mcg/ml. Side-effects of theophylline are less likely to occur if the dose is built up slowly. A reasonable starting dose is around 7 mg/kg/day increased after a week if there are no side-effects. In adults a convenient starting dose is 200 mg twice a day. Because of the different slow-release mechanisms it is not possible to interchange different commercial preparations without rechecking the blood levels. The blood level provides a check on compliance with therapy. Many patients do not take their treatment as prescribed and this can lead to a problem when patients are admitted to hospital and given their drugs under supervision (Fig. 9.3). The prescribed dose, when actually taken, may produce side-effects which were not evident at home because of the missed doses.

Anti-leukotrienes

Anti-leukotrienes need to be taken orally. The absorption of the leukotriene receptor antagonist zafirlukast is affected by food and it needs to be taken an hour before or more than two hours after meals. This is not a problem with zilueton which inhibits 5-lipoxygenase. This is through inhibition of microsomal CYP3A4 enzyme; metabolism of drugs such as theophylline, terfenadine and warfarin may be affected and the doses should be adjusted.

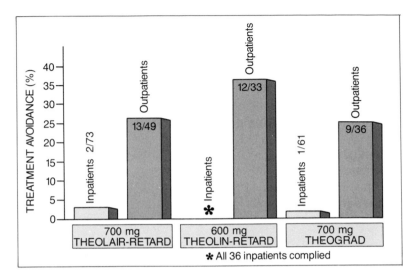

Figure 9.3 Percentage and number of patients with no detectable plasma theophylline concentration (in- and outpatients are shown separately). Twenty-nine per cent of outpatients were not taking their prescribed treatment.

Corticosteroids

In a small proportion of asthmatics long-term oral corticosteroids will be necessary (see Chapter 5). There was a suggestion that the adverse effects associated with steroids, such as osteoporosis, might be less common in asthma but this has been shown to be untrue.[21] Therefore, it is important to keep the dose as low as possible while retaining the desired effect. Prednisolone is the drug usually chosen and there is no advantage in using longer-acting steroids such as betamethasone, dexamethasone or depot preparations. The prednisolone is best given as a single daily dose in the morning.

Unwanted effects can be minimized by the use of alternate day treatment and by using concomitant inhaled steroids to restrict the oral prednisolone dose. It is not unusual for alternate day therapy to produce inadequate control of asthma on the day off treatment. Patients vary but, generally, hypothalamus–pituitary–adrenal (HPA) axis suppression is seen above a dose of 7.5 mg prednisolone per day.

Side-effects   There are few problems with side-effects when using a short course of steroids for acute exacerbations. Most likely to occur are:

- Fluid retention
- Precipitation of diabetes mellitus
- Gastric irritation
- Steroid psychosis

With long-term treatment the following familiar side-effects present a problem:

- Truncal obesity
- Protein wasting
- Osteoporosis
- Cataracts
- Stunting of growth in children

Fluid retention is less troublesome with methylprednisolone which should be used if oedema or heart failure has been a problem with previous courses. With long-term oral steroids a check should be kept on the electrolytes for hypokalaemia. Those patients who have problems with indigestion from oral corticosteroids may be helped by the use of enteric-coated prednisolone. There is no advantage in the use of ACTH by injection, since suppression of the HPA axis still occurs, but at a pituitary rather than an adrenal level.

INJECTION

Beta$_2$ agonists

Subcutaneous adrenaline was once a regular form of treatment in acute asthma. But with the advent of selective agents, adrenaline is no longer necessary. Treatment with nebulized drugs provides just as good a response as subcutaneous or intravenous injection. Thus there are few circumstances where such treatment is necessary.

Intravenous salbutamol or terbutaline can be used by continuous infusion for the treatment of severe acute asthma. They may have a place where nebulized therapy appears not to be working. This may occur when a lot of mucus plugging is present, restricting penetration by the inhaled route.[102]

Occasional asthmatic patients who are known to have sudden catastrophic exacerbations may benefit from carrying injectable beta$_2$ agonists with them. Such patients may progress from good control to life-threatening asthma within an hour or so. They can be taught to administer 0.25 mg terbutaline or salbutamol subcutaneously to themselves in such an emergency.

Careful explanation and practice is needed if such an emergency treatment is going to be carried and used successfully during a severe exacerbation. Relatives should be instructed also so that they can help in a crisis.

Occasional patients have such poor control of their asthma that the use of continuous subcutaneous infusion of beta$_2$ agonist is justified. A "butterfly" needle is inserted subcutaneously, usually on the abdomen, and connected to a small portable pump carried in a pouch on a belt. Doses of around 10–20 mg (10–20 ml) terbutaline in 24 hours are typical. Blood levels of terbutaline are high and this treatment should be reserved for extreme problems. The injection site lasts 1–3 days on average. Patients learn to place their own needle and adjust their pump. Infections and subcutaneous nodules at injection sites are an occasional problem. After months or years on such treatment patients may be able to discontinue their pump and resort to more conventional treatment.

Aminophylline

The ethylenediamine salt of theophylline, aminophylline, is more soluble and is used for intravenous therapy. With intravenous aminophylline the same problems of variation in rate of metabolism and poor safety margin occur as with oral therapy (discussed previously). The initial loading dose of aminophylline must be given slowly, over fifteen minutes. Injecting at this slow pace is quite difficult in practice and is most easily given diluted in normal saline in a paediatric burette.

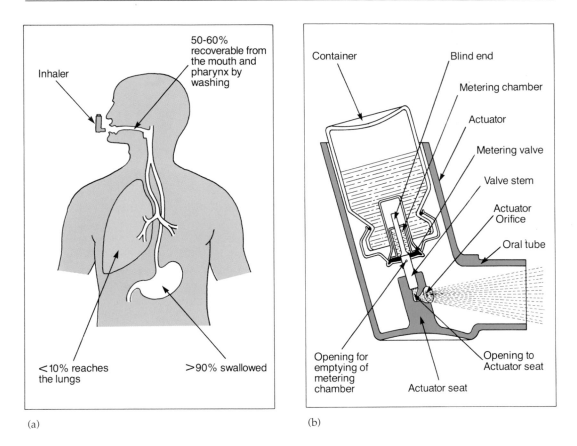

Figure 9.4 (a) Distribution of the output of the metered dose inhaler. (b) Metered dose inhaler mechanism.

INHALED ROUTE

Metered dose inhalers

Beta$_2$ agonists, anticholinergic agents and corticosteroids are frequently prescribed in metered dose inhalers (Fig. 9.4). Particles inhaled through the mouth have to turn a corner to enter the respiratory tract through the larynx. The particles leaving a metered dose inhaler do so with considerable velocity and many of them impact in the oropharynx. This is more likely with larger, heavier particles and faster particles. Even with a perfect technique of inhalation only about 10 per cent of the dose leaving the inhaler reaches the respiratory tract. Ninety per cent is deposited in the mouth and subsequently swallowed.[103] The dose then absorbed from the gastrointestinal tract is too low to produce therapeutic or toxic effects.

Metered dose inhalers have the advantage that they are familiar to many asthmatics and that they are cheaper than newer devices. Current inhalers contain fluorocarbons which contribute a very small proportion of the fluorocarbons released into the atmosphere each year. Some countries have banned their use or set restrictions on the current inhalers. The use of these will be banned in the UK in the next few years. Pharmaceutical companies are now reformulating their pressurized inhalers with new non-CFC propellants.

A small number of youngsters misuse their inhalers to obtain a general sympathomimetic effect. This problem can usually be dealt with by switching to a dry powder system.

Teaching inhaler technique   The use of various inhaler devices requires some skill on the part of the patient (Fig. 9.5). Teaching the correct method of use is an essential part of the prescription of such treatment. The technique of inhalation should be checked each time the patient is seen until both parties are confident that this is being done correctly. After this periodic review is advisable.

Many patients will need to have the advice repeated over a number of visits before they become competent. Failure to master a metered dose inhaler occurs in many patients at all ages. Problems are even more common in older subjects. The minority of patients who never manage to cope with a metered dose inhaler can almost always be taught to use one of the alternative devices. The instructions issued by manufacturers vary and are not all correct. The essential features are:

1. **Shake the canister**   This disperses the drug uniformly throughout the propellants. It also allows the patient to confirm that the canister is not empty.
2. **Position**   The canister should be held upright and directed into the mouth. If it is not upright the metering chamber will not refill and the next actuation will produce a reduced output.

   It has been shown that keeping the mouth wide open and holding the inhaler several centimetres away provides more lung deposition.[104] This works by allowing the cloud of particles to slow down before impacting in the mouth and allows evaporation of propellant to obtain a smaller size of particle. However, this does make the technique more difficult and makes it more likely that the aerosol cloud will miss the mouth altogether. Therefore, it is not recommended except in very co-operative patients.
3. **Timing**   The drug will be effective only if it is breathed in during inspiration. About one-third of patients initially have trouble with this coordination. A frequent problem when inhalers are first used is that the shock of the cold spray reaching the pharynx abruptly stops inspiration. The problem usually resolves as the patient becomes familiar with the sensation.

   There is some controversy about the lung volume at which the actuation should occur.[105] It probably makes little difference whether this is done at low lung volume when there is more inspiratory flow to follow, or at high lung volume when the airways are wider, but it is simpler to teach patients to discharge the inhaler at the beginning of an inspiration.

   One frequent mistake in those asked to take two puffs regularly is to try to take both puffs during the same inhalation. Only one actuation should occur per breath.
4. **Speed of inspiration**   The flow rate of inspiration should be slow.[106] This decreases impaction in the pharynx and produces deeper penetration into the airways, since

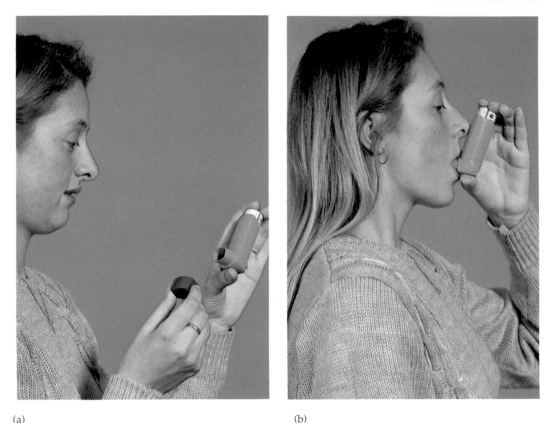

(a)   (b)

Figure 9.5 Metered dose inhaler technique.
(a) The patient removes the cap and shakes the inhaler.
(b) Actuation should be towards the start of a slow deep inspiration.

flow is laminar rather than turbulent. This is contrary to some of the manufacturers' instructions.

5. **Breath holding**   At the end of slow, deep inspiration, the patient should hold his or her breath to allow any particles still suspended in the airways to settle. Ideally the breath should be held for ten seconds.

6. **The next dose**   Theoretically, if the drug being inhaled is a bronchodilator, it is desirable to wait for the bronchodilatation to occur before taking the next dose. This would allow the second dose to get to the airways the first dose could not reach. This complicates the procedure and is not usually recommended unless airflow obstruction is quite marked. Similarly there seems to be no benefit in routinely waiting ten minutes after a bronchodilator aerosol before taking an inhaled corticosteroid.[107]

Patients need to be aware of when their inhaler is getting close to empty. Test firing in the air is one way but wastes a large number of doses unnecessarily. Most patients can

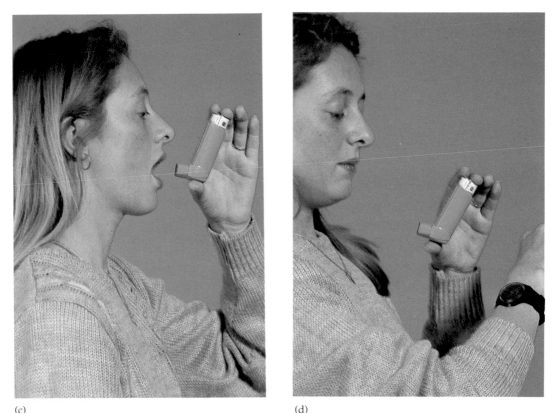

(c)   (d)

(c) Responses may be better when the inhaler is actuated an inch or two away from the open mouth but there is more room for error with this technique.
(d) After the full inspiration the breath should be held for five to ten seconds.

be taught to tell by shaking their inhaler. It has been suggested that placing the chamber in water may be helpful by the fact that the chamber floats symmetrically upright when close to empty. Patients need to become aware of the supply left in their inhaler to avoid being caught in an exacerbation without adequate relief.

Beta$_2$ agonists

New devices for inhalation are being developed regularly, but those currently available are listed in the table on page 126.

Extension tubes and spacer devices[108]

Short extension tubes such as the spacer on the terbutaline metered dose inhaler provide some help for patients with poor coordination. However, large volume spacing devices such as the Nebuhaler and the Volumatic provide the best method to separate the timing

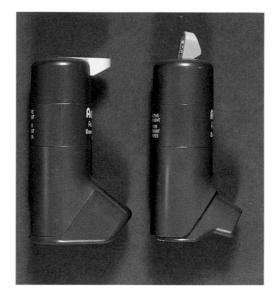

Figure 9.6 Breath-actuated inhaler.

of the firing of the inhaler from inspiration. These 750 ml plastic chambers allow small particles to stay in suspension and evaporation of the propellant produces more particles of respirable size. Inspiration should be as soon as possible after firing the inhaler; delays reduce the drug available for inspiration. If the inhaler is fired more than once then there is a comparative loss of drug delivered. For two inhalations the loss is small (perhaps 20 per cent) but with more firings the loss is substantial. The recently introduced Babyhaler with a volume of 350 ml can be used by infants and small children.

Spacing devices increase lung deposition to 20–30 per cent. They virtually remove oropharyngeal deposition. This is most important for inhaled corticosteroids where the incidence of oral thrush and dysphonia is reduced. The small amount of gastrointestinal absorption will not occur reducing the potential for systemic effects to drug absorbed from the lungs.

During acute exacerbations of asthma coordination with inhaled devices will be more difficult and inspiratory airflow too low for efficient lung penetration. The spacing devices can be used as a means of delivering bronchodilators as an alternative to a nebulizer in acute episodes or for chronic therapy. Even young children can use them with the aid of a facemask fitted to the end of the spacer.

The spacers should be taken apart and cleaned about once a week. They are suitable for home use although too bulky to carry around easily. Static charge builds up on spacer devices; this attracts drug particles and reduces drug delivery. This is reduced by washing the spacer but gradually builds up again. Spacers carried by nurses or doctors for occasional use should also be washed regularly.

Breath-actuated metered dose inhalers

Breath-actuated devices are primed before actuation and the metered dose inhaler is triggered by inspiratory airflow (Fig. 9.6). The airflow required is low and the triggering

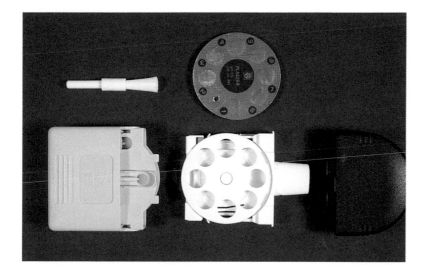

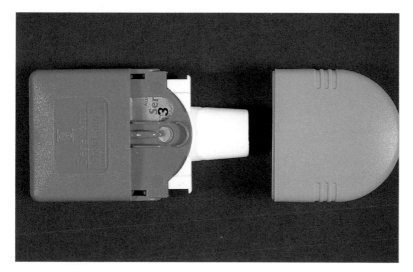

Figure 9.7 The Diskhaler.

of the device quiet enough not to disturb the inspiration. These devices are now available for beta$_2$ agonists, anticholinergics, corticosteroids and sodium cromoglycate so that patients who find this form of inhaler best can use it for all their inhaled treatment.

Dry powder systems

a)   Diskhaler (Fig. 9.7)

The dry powder disk system has four or eight doses in one disk. Each dose is sealed to prevent problems with humidity. The system is easy to use and available for treatment with salbutamol, salmeterol, beclomethasone dipropionate and fluticasone propionate.

b)   Turbohaler (Fig. 9.8)
     The Turbohaler is a multidose dry powder system which is available for terbutaline
     and budesonide. The drug is present without any carrier. It requires an inspiratory
     airflow of only 60 l/min in order to produce lung deposition around 20 per cent.
     Some patients find that the lack of sensation from the powder is disturbing. Most
     patients find the system easy to use.

c)   Diskus/Accuhaler
     The Diskus/Accuhaler is a dry powder multidose system providing up to one
     month's treatment. It is available initially as salmeterol and fluticasone propionate.
     Each dose is sealed to prevent problems with humidity.

d)   Rotacaps
     The original dry powder system for salbutamol and beclomethasone dipropionate
     was the Rotahaler (Figs 9.9 and 9.10). Each dose has to be loaded individually into
     the Rotahaler. The lactose powder in the capsule may cause coughing. The deliv-
     ery into the lung from the Rotahaler is probably much the same as that from the
     metered dose inhaler. Rotacaps need to be kept in a dry place. If they are exposed
     to moisture or to extremes of temperature then the particles clump together and
     become too large to inhale.

Selective beta$_2$ agonists by inhalation

	Metered dose inhaler (mdi)		Other
	Dose per actuation	Doses per inhaler	
• Salbutamol	100 mcg	200	Rotacaps (dry powder) 200 mcg and 400 mcg. Ventodisks (dry powder) 200 mcg and 400 mcg. Aerolin Autohaler 100 mcg. Cyclocaps (dry powder) 200 mcg and 400 mcg + Cyclohaler mdi + volumatic.
• Terbutaline	250 mcg	400	mdi + spacer mdi + Nebuhaler Turbohaler (dry powder) 500 mcg, 100 doses
• Fenoterol	100, 200 mcg	200	-
• Pirbuterol	200 mcg	200	-
• Reproterol	500 mcg	400	-
• Rimiterol	200 mcg	300	-
• Salmeterol	25 mcg	120	Diskhaler 50 mcg, Accuhaler 50 mcg

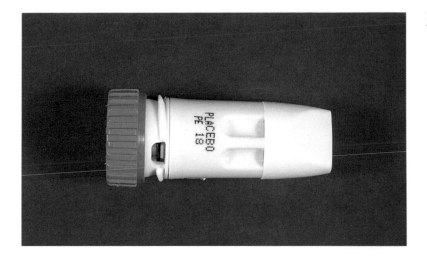

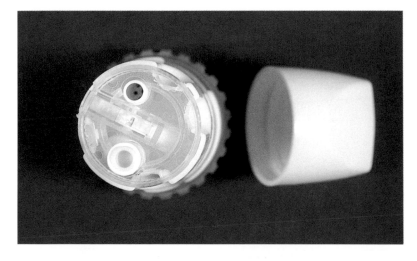

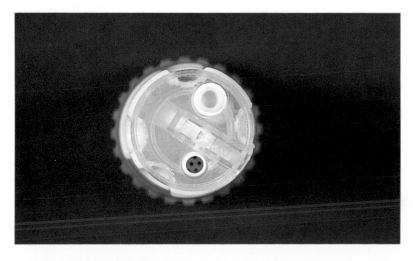

Figure 9.8 The Turbohaler.

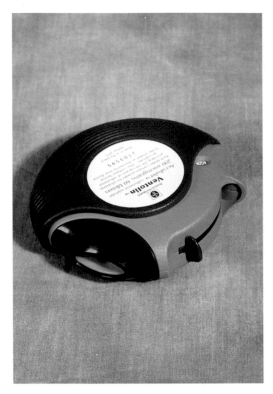

Figure 9.9 The Accuhaler.

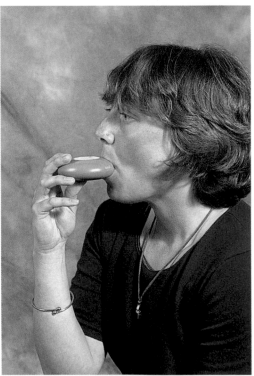

Figure 9.10 The Accuhaler in use.

Nebulizers

Nebulizers can be used for the administration of:

- Beta$_2$ agonists
- Ipratropium bromide
- Sodium cromoglycate
- Budesonide

Airway narrowing in acute asthma may limit inspiratory airflow to such an extent that metered dose inhalers cannot be taken into the lungs well enough to be effective. In these circumstances nebulization will still be effective, as only tidal breathing is necessary. In acute asthma nebulized beta$_2$ agonists produce as good a response as intravenous therapy.

How they work   Most nebulizers available are of the jet type, where a high-velocity stream of air or oxygen sucks liquid up a tube by the Venturi principle. This liquid is broken into particles at an opening at the top of the tube (Fig. 9.11).

Ultrasonic nebulizers are also available (Fig. 9.12). In these a piezo-electric transducer produces high-frequency waves. Small surface waves are produced which rupture and release small droplets.

How to use them   Nebulizers only perform adequately if proper attention is given to the details of their use. These vary with the type of nebulizer used. Most nebulizers leave behind approximately 1 ml of the solution added to them in the apparatus itself. Therefore the larger the volume to which the nebulized drug is diluted, the smaller will be the amount of active drug left behind. However, increasing the volume also increases the time necessary for nebulization. In practice a volume of 4 ml is a good compromise in most nebulizers.

Newer chambers have baffle arrangements to conserve nebulizer solution or arrangements to divert flow away from the chamber during expiration reducing wastage into the atmosphere while the patient is breathing out. Such devices may allow a smaller amount of drug to be used.

The flow rate of gas through the nebulizer affects the time taken and the particle size of the nebulizer output. For maximal deposition in the lungs the particle size (mass median diameter) should be 2-5 μm.[109] Above 10 μm few particles get beyond the oropharynx.

A flow rate of 6 l/min is needed to nebulize 4 ml solution in around ten minutes or less. Flow rates of 4 l/min double the time required. For the particle size to be in the required range a flow rate of 8 l/min is desirable.[110]

Either air or oxygen can be used as a driving gas for jet nebulizers.[111] At home air is simplest to use because air compressors will produce a suitable flow rate. Domiciliary oxygen supplies only produce 4 l/min on their highest setting and so they are not adequate to power jet nebulizers. Alternative fittings can be supplied and serviced from hospitals but the cylinders used at home very quickly run out at a flow rate of 8 l/min. Light, portable compressors are particularly useful for travelling (Figure 9.13). For occasional use a simple footpump has proved useful.

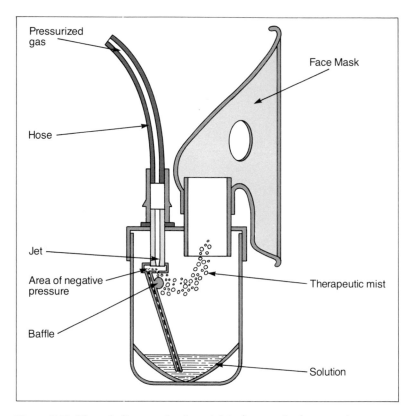

Figure 9.11 The nebulizer mechanism. A jet of pressurized gas creates an area of negative pressure causing the solution to rise from the well. When it reaches the area of negative pressure it is bombarded by the jet of gas and broken up into a mist which leaves the outlet, as an aerosol, directed towards the patient. Larger particles hit the baffle and fall back into the well.

Dangers with nebulizers   There are theoretical dangers with each driving gas. Oxygen may produce problems in chronic airflow obstruction with CO_2 retention which may worsen on breathing oxygen. Using air as the driving gas is potentially dangerous in acute asthma. Patients are already hypoxic and bronchodilators may occasionally worsen this. They relax smooth muscle in pulmonary blood vessels, thus returning blood flow to hypoventilated areas where local hypoxia has induced constriction. This is an uncommon finding.

Oxygen should be used as the driving gas in acute asthma or continued by nasal prongs during an air driven nebulization.

Anticholinergic agents

The two anticholinergic agents available in the UK are ipratropium bromide (Fig. 9.14) and oxitropium bromide. Oxitropium has a longer duration of action allowing twice or three times daily use. The onset of action is slower than that for beta$_2$ agonists,

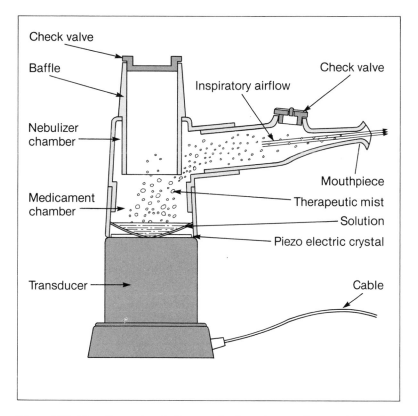

Figure 9.12 The ultrasonic nebulizer mechanism. A resonating crystal sends a series of waves through the solution. This creates a "cone" of solution from which small particles break off to form a mist which is then inhaled by the patient.

taking thirty to sixty minutes to reach its maximal effect, but the length of action is greater than conventional short-acting beta$_2$ agonists such as salbutamol and terbutaline.

Anticholinergic agents are available as metered dose inhalers and as breath-actuated metered dose inhalers in the UK. In some countries dry powder systems are marketed. Ipratropium bromide is available as a nebulizer solution. The metered dose inhaler is also available as a combined preparation with fenoterol or salbutamol. It has been suggested that fenoterol was involved in the rise in asthma deaths in New Zealand in the 1980s and that it may have more cardiostimulatory activity than other selective beta$_2$ agonists. However, it has been marketed now as a lower dose inhaler (100 mcg rather than 200 mcg), the same dose as the combined preparation. In general, fixed-dose preparations are best avoided in a variable condition such as asthma unless it is thought that they will significantly improve compliance.

There is some suggestion that the dose of ipratropium bromide in the conventional inhaler may be too low (20 mcg) for some patients and a higher strength inhaler (40 mcg) is available. Higher doses of anticholinergic agents are not associated with significant side-effects.

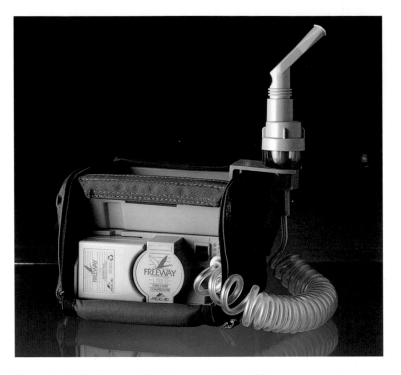

Figure 9.13 The Freeway Lite Luxury Nebulizer/Compressor system.

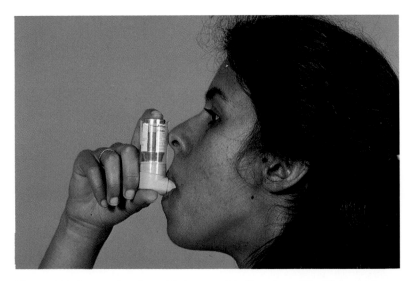

Figure 9.14 Ipratropium bromide is an anticholinergic agent which may be particularly useful in older patients and very young children. The onset of action is slower than with beta$_2$ agonists but the duration of action may be a little longer.

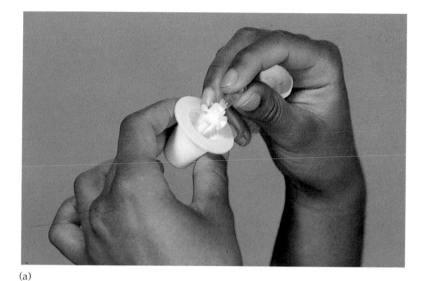

(a)

(b)

Figure 9.15 Spinhaler technique.
(a) The sodium cromoglycate capsule is inserted into the Spinhaler.
(b) Moving the collar of the Spinhaler allows two metal prongs to pierce the capsule. (Continued overleaf.)

Sodium cromoglycate and nedocromil sodium

For a number of years sodium cromoglycate has been available as a dry powder inhalation by means of Spincaps in a Spinhaler (Figs 9.15 and 9.16). There are plain Spinhalers or a combined preparation which contains 100 mcg isoprenaline in addition to 20 mg sodium cromoglycate. A combined preparation with salbutamol is also available.

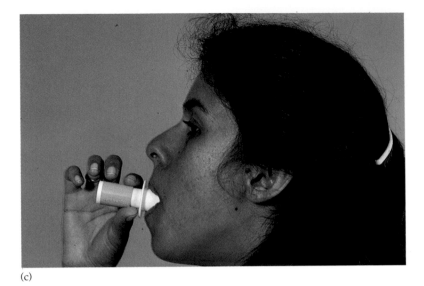

(c)

Figure 9.15 Spinhaler technique (continued).
(c) Sodium cromoglycate powder is inhaled with a deep inspiration. This may
need to be repeated to empty the capsule completely.

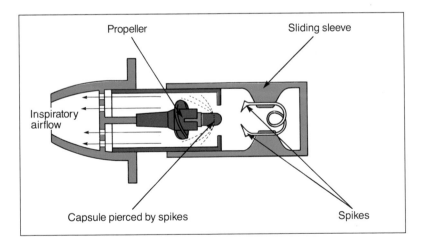

Figure 9.16 The mechanism of the sodium cromoglycate Spinhaler. The
propeller is spun by the inspiratory airflow. This rotates the capsule and
powder emerges through holes previously made by the spikes.

The compound capsules are designed to counteract the bronchoconstriction which
occasionally follows the inhalation of dry powder. Because the isoprenaline component
produces bronchodilatation there is a tendency for the compound capsules to be used
inappropriately for symptomatic relief, rather than regularly as prophylaxis. Therefore,
they are best avoided. Patients who do wheeze with the dry powder can take a $beta_2$
agonist just before the cromoglycate, or switch to the metered dose inhaler.

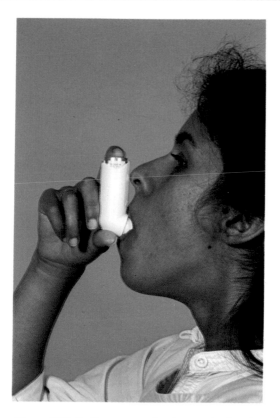

Figure 9.17 Sodium cromoglycate can also be given by metered dose inhaler.

Metered dose inhalers of sodium cromoglycate (Fig. 9.17) provide 5 mg per actuation and are usually given as two inhalations four times a day. This may be lowered to one four times daily for maintenance treatment.

Sodium cromoglycate is available as a breath-actuated metered dose inhaler, as a nebulizer solution and with a 700 ml chamber spacer device (Fisonair).

Nedocromil sodium has a bitter taste which some patients find unpleasant. This is disguised by mint flavouring in the metered dose inhaler which is produced with a small spacing device as an option (Fig. 9.18).

Corticosteroids

Three corticosteroid preparations are available in Britain (see table overleaf). They are usually given twice daily. The only significant side-effects of inhaled corticosteroids in conventional doses are oropharyngeal candidiasis and hoarseness. Candidiasis occurs in around 5 per cent of patients but is more common at higher doses (Fig. 9.19).[112] Some degree of hoarseness unrelated to candida is more common, but the actual incidence varies greatly between studies.

The hoarseness may be related to a local myopathy of the vocal cords and improves on stopping the steroids.[113]

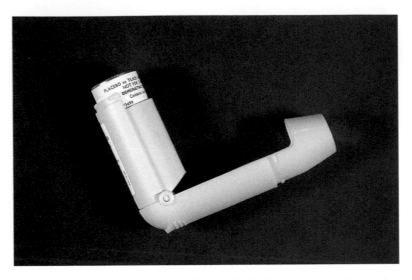

Figure 9.18 The Syncroner device is designed to help overcome problems of coordination in inhalation. It is available for sodium cromoglycate and nedocromil sodium.

Corticosteroids for inhalation

Preparation	Form	Dose per actuation	Doses per inhaler
● Beclomethasone dipropionate	Metered dose inhaler (standard)	50, 100 and 200 mcg	200
	Metered dose inhaler (high-dose)	250 mcg	200
	Diskhaler	100, 200 and 400 mcg	8
	Rotacaps	100 mcg (paediatric) 200 and 400 mcg (adult)	
	Breath-actuated metered dose inhaler	50, 100 and 250 mcg	200
	Nebulizer solution	50 mcg/ml (paediatric)	
● Budesonide	Metered dose inhaler + collapsible spacer	200 mcg (adult) 50 mcg (paediatric)	100 200
	Turbohaler	100 mcg 200 mcg 400 mcg	200 100 50
	Nebulizer solution	250 mcg/ml or 500 mcg/ml	
● Fluticasone proprionate	Diskhaler	50, 100, 250 and 500 mcg	4
	Metered dose inhaler	25, 50, 125 and 250 mcg	120
	Accuhaler	50, 100, 250 and 500 mcg	

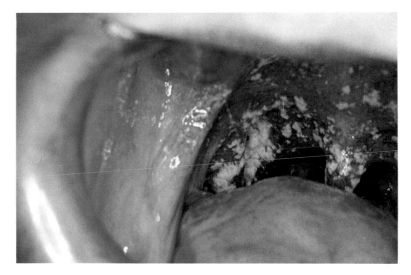

Figure 9.19 Candidiasis is a side-effect of conventional doses of inhaled corticosteroids in around 5 per cent of patients.

Beclomethasone dipropionate can be used as a metered dose inhaler. At doses above 800 mcg daily a large volume spacer should be used to reduce oral candida and dysphonia. Alternative breath-actuated devices are available.

Budesonide Budesonide is supplied with a collapsible spacer similar to that used for terbutaline (Fig. 9.20). Subsequent prescriptions need be only for the refill canister. The spacer might reduce oropharyngeal deposition and candida in the mouth, but not the incidence of hoarseness. It can be given with a spacing chamber or by the dry powder Turbohaler system.

Budesonide is the only corticosteroid available as a nebulizer solution in a dose suitable for adults.

Fluticasone propionate is a new inhaled steroid which seems to have a greater local action and less likelihood of systemic problems. It is effective at half the equivalent dose to beclomethasone dipropionate. At present it is available as a metered dose inhaler and Accuhaler and Diskhaler dry powder system. It should certainly be considered when doses of inhaled steroid reach 1,000 mcg.

Dosage As doses of inhaled corticosteroids are increased, an effect on the HPA axis becomes demonstrable. However, up to a dose of 1,600 mcg beclomethasone dipropionate per day, or its equivalent, there is no evidence of clinically important adrenal

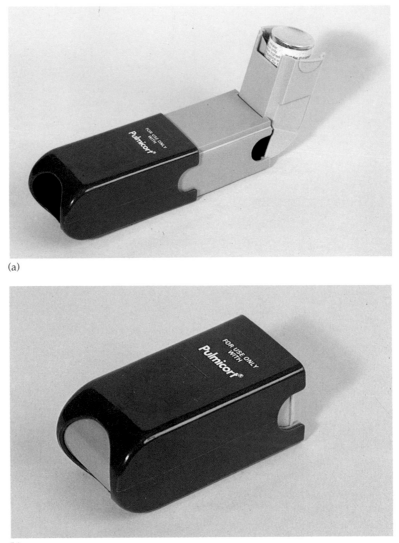

(a)

(b)

Figure 9.20 (a) The spacer mechanism is available for use with terbutaline and budesonide. It partly overcomes the problems of coordination with metered dose inhalers. (b) This spacer collapses into a device no bigger than a simple metered dose inhaler.

suppression in adults. At doses above 1,000 mcg daily skin thinning and purpura is possible. Biochemical effects on bone formation can be demonstrated, but there has been no convincing evidence of osteoporosis from inhaled steroids at these doses. At doses of inhaled steroids above 1000 mcg daily beclomethasone (or equivalent), general measures to reduce the risk of osteoporosis should be reviewed. These include regular exercise, adequate calcium intake and hormone replacement where appropriate. Systemic absorption can be reduced by rinsing the mouth and spitting out the contents after inhaler use.

PRACTICAL POINTS

- It is good practice to try routinely to use inhaled therapy for asthma. This keeps the dose down and reduces side-effects.

- With the wide range of devices available most patients can be taught to use inhaled treatment.

- The patient should be given detailed instructions on the correct way to use an inhaler, with regular follow-up to check technique.

- In severe asthma, inspiratory flow may not be adequate for metered dose inhalers. In this situation a nebulizer or large volume spacer is required for inhaled treatment.

10
Physical and psychological treatments

Physiotherapy

In acute severe exacerbations of asthma physiotherapists are often involved in the administration of drugs by nebulizers. Since they are familiar with the equipment this helps to ensure that the nebulizers are used to their best advantage. When sputum retention is a problem, physiotherapy can help the patients to cough up tenacious plugs of mucus (Fig. 10.1). When there is plentiful mucus in the airways its removal by physiotherapy improves airflow obstruction.

Exercise to keep fit can be recommended for most patients, asthmatic or not. Fit patients ventilate less at a given workload and this will increase the threshold for the development of exercise-induced asthma (see Chapter 3).

Breathing exercises have been used for many years in the management of asthma but they are still a controversial subject. There is no good scientific evidence to support their use. It seems unlikely that a very breathless patient fighting for breath during a severe exacerbation will be able to control his breathing as he has been taught, though this is not to say that breathing exercises cannot be helpful.

Some patients tend to panic easily, and when they begin to wheeze they may then markedly hyperventilate and so increase their airflow obstruction. They may also then be unable to coordinate their breathing to use inhaled therapy in this state. Concentration on rhythmic patterns of breathing which they have been previously taught may let them relax, stop hyperventilating, take their inhaled therapy and prevent the downward trend in their asthma.

Bronchial lavage

Bronchial lavage has been used in the treatment of acute and chronic asthma. The rationale for its use in acute asthma is the removal of the mucus plugs which the patients may be unable to cough up. This is certainly not a routine treatment in this situation. Most physicians regard it as a desperate measure to be turned to when an asthmatic continues to present problems after being placed on a ventilator.

A simple form of lavage consists of injecting fluid down an endotracheal tube and then aspirating it back. A formal lavage consists of isolating a lobe or segment with a

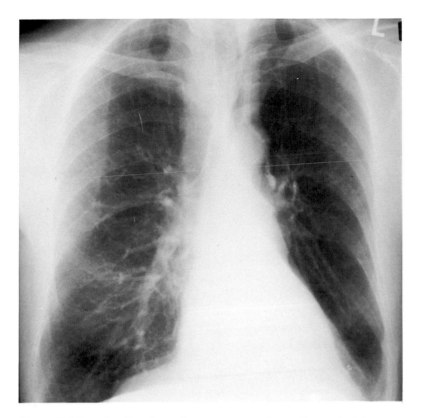

Figure 10.1 Occasionally, plugs of mucus may produce collapse of a lobe or whole lung. This chest X-ray shows collapse of the left lower lobe. Physiotherapy may then be helpful to stimulate coughing and reinflate the collapsed areas.

specialized endotracheal tube, or by wedging the fibreoptic bronchoscope. Large quantities of fluid are then instilled into the isolated area, hoping to free the mucus plugs and suck them out.

Ionizers

Some manufacturers have made considerable claims of the benefits to be obtained from the use of air ionizers. With only a slightly higher ratio of positive ions at ground level, very few charged particles are normally present in the air. Various factors such as humidity and dust may affect this.

Ionizers provide negatively charged particles by passing air over electrostatically charged plates. Short-term exposure does not change lung function. Studies of exposure to ionized air at night for some weeks suggest a small effect in a few patients.[114] There may also be a reduction in exercise-induced bronchoconstriction when inspired air contains one hundred times the normal concentration of ionized particles.[115]

The way in which such an effect might be brought about is unclear. It has been suggested that negatively ionized air increases the metabolism of 5-hydroxy-tryptamine.[116] 5-Hydroxytryptamine may produce bronchoconstriction when inhaled but there is no evidence that it is an important mediator in asthma. Any response to ionizers is considerably smaller than the response to conventional pharmacological treatment.

Acupuncture

This technique has long been used in China for the management of asthma. Various relevant points have been described, such as Tiantu (Ren channel No. 22 in the suprasternal notch), Dingchuan (extra point 17, 1.2 cm either side of the seventh cervical vertebra) and Lieque (lung channel No 7, 5 cm proximal to the styloid process of the radius). One study of these three points showed no overall benefit, while at the same time a control group using nonspecific points Xuanli and Xaunlu (in the temporal hairline) improved![61]

Another small study using point Dingchuan (see above) found no changes in baseline lung function but suggested an increased bronchodilator response to salbutamol.[117] None of these studies suggests that acupuncture has an important place in the treatment of asthma.

Hypnosis

This has been used for many years in the treatment of asthma but there have been few scientific attempts to assess its effect. One controlled study of one year's treatment with hypnosis compared to breathing exercises found no significant difference between the two.[62]

Hypnosis can change the perception of asthma so that patients may feel better even though objective tests of airflow obstruction are unchanged. It may also reduce the bronchoconstrictor response to exercise in some patients. Similar effects can be produced by simple suggestion or administration of a placebo. However, these responses are small compared to the effects of pretreatment with inhaled sodium cromoglycate or beta$_2$ agonists.

Relaxation

In some trials, interventions such as yoga have provided some benefit in the control of asthma. It is difficult to produce adequately controlled trials in many of these areas. Asthma produces anxiety and in acute exacerbations it is the asthma itself which needs to be relieved, not the anxiety. However, anxiety can worsen asthma and confidence in dealing with problems can lead to a general improvement.

PRACTICAL POINTS

- Physiotherapy can help to remove tenacious mucus plugs from the airways.
- Simple rhythmic breathing exercises may help agitated patients to stop hyper-ventilating and to use their inhaled therapy more effectively.
- Bronchial lavage is a last-ditch measure, reserved for patients who fail to respond to ventilator therapy.
- The beneficial effects on asthma of ionizers, acupuncture and hypnosis are insignificant compared with modern drug treatments.

11
Patient education

This final chapter is intended to deal with some day-to-day practical questions patients often have about schooling, exercise, jobs, and the like in relation to their asthma. Such information is part of the education of patients about the management of their condition. This education is often neglected by practitioners but is vitally important in dealing with asthma. Most asthmatics lead a virtually normal life, not significantly affected by their disease; but a few, despite optimal treatment, have persistent symptoms. And some patients find it helpful to obtain information by association with other patients in organizations such as the National Asthma Campaign in Britain. Useful addresses can be found in the appendix.

School

Absence   Asthma is responsible for a large proportion of absences from school. In some cases this is because it has not been recognized and is being inappropriately treated as bronchitis with antibiotics, rather than bronchodilators. With effective treatment the great majority lose very little time from school. A study of thirty-one asthmatic children found that starting prophylactic treatment reduced school absences tenfold. There has been a suggestion that, on average, asthmatic children are brighter than normal. Certainly they are not less intelligent.

Games   Sport often produces problems. Here again most asthmatics have few difficulties if they take adequate treatment before exercise (see page 33). They can usually participate normally. Sports such as swimming may be more suitable than those such as cross-country running, where prolonged exercise in cold air is necessary. Teachers must be put fully in the picture so that they appreciate the needs and treatment of asthmatic children. With young children they may need to be involved in the administration of treatment during the day. The National Asthma Campaign have information packs available for school nurses and teachers.

Special schools and environments   There are a few asthmatic children who have such problems at ordinary schools that their education begins to suffer. In Britain, when this happens, special day or residential schools are available. These schools produce their own particular problems by grouping together children in an abnormal environment. They should be considered only when it is felt that prolonged absences from school could be avoided by the skills of teachers at a special school.

Removal to environments such as centres in Switzerland often improves asthma. However, there is very little long-term benefit to be gained from these excursions as on return to the home surroundings symptoms recur just as before.

Need for normality   Every effort should be made to get children to live as normal a life as possible. This is helped by explanation of the treatment and outlook to patient and parents. Many children will grow out of their asthma (see Chapter 2) and the aim should be to prepare them all for a normal adult life by conventional schooling and activity, made possible by suitable supervision and therapy.

Exercise

There is no evidence that exercise is harmful for asthmatics. It may produce transient bronchoconstriction but this is easily dealt with. Such reactions are less likely to occur as patients become fitter since they can achieve the same goals with less ventilation and, therefore, less airway cooling. Beta$_2$ agonists are the most successful agents in preventing exercise-induced bronchoconstriction. Sodium cromoglycate is also usually effective, but ipratropium bromide much less so.

Warming-up   Although there are no good trials to prove it, many doctors involved with exercise and asthma are convinced of the benefit of a warm-up period before strenuous exercise. Warm-up periods make pulled muscles less likely and significantly improve the performance of normal subjects, and they are particularly advisable for asthmatic athletes.[118]

Drug regulations   Recent changes in regulations have ensured that competitive athletes may take adequate treatment to control their asthma. Sodium cromoglycate, inhaled steroids, and the selective beta$_2$ agonists, oral and inhaled, are all allowed. The nonselective agents such as ephedrine and isoprenaline are banned by the International Olympic Committee. In competitive international sports where tests for drug use are employed, it is still wise to inform the authorities of the need for treatment, even when this is permitted.

Diet

There are no problems with diet in asthma, except in a few patients with specific food sensitivities (see Chapter 3). So unless such sensitivities have been identified, asthmatics can eat what they like. However, they should avoid becoming overweight as this increases the work of breathing.

Occupations

The problems of occupational asthma, now a legally recognized industrial disease in Britain, are discussed in Chapter 3. Atopic subjects without asthma may be advised to avoid jobs where a high degree of sensitization is known to occur, such as in metal-refining or detergent industries. However, environmental control is preferable to such restrictions.

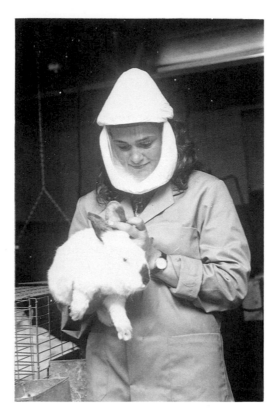

Figure 11.1 When asthmatic patients have to continue working in an environment containing inhaled allergens to which they are sensitive, a mask and filtered air system can provide very useful protection.

Asthmatics with more than mild symptoms should avoid jobs where they may be exposed to extremes of climate or to a great deal of dust or irritant fumes - building work, for example. However, asthmatics are to be found working quite happily in almost all jobs. In some situations where difficulties do arise, such as workers with small laboratory animals, it may be possible to avoid problems by the use of suitable masks to filter inspired air (Fig. 11.1).

Asthma in women

Pregnancy   As discussed in Chapter 3, the course of asthma during pregnancy is difficult to predict. Approximately one-third of asthmatics have a deterioration of their asthma, while one-third improve. There are obviously worries about the effect on the fetus of any drugs administered to control asthma, but the fetus is more likely to be at risk from uncontrolled asthma and from hypoxia than from the treatment.

Beta$_2$ agonists are thought to be safe in the treatment of asthma in pregnancy. During pregnancy there is even more reason than usual for using inhaled therapy to keep the dose of drug down. Theophyllines are also safe. Corticosteroids should be used as necessary. Animal studies suggesting an increased in cleft lip and palate in animals given steroids have not been confirmed in humans.

Steroid-dependent asthmatics should be given hydrocortisone to cover the delivery but there appears to be no need to give corticosteroids to the baby after delivery.

If antibiotics are given, then tetracyclines should, of course, be avoided in pregnancy.

Menstruation   Asthma may show cyclical variation with menstruation. Subjective changes with menstruation seem to occur more commonly than can be shown on objective measurements, and there is some evidence that perception of the degree of airflow obstruction may vary with the menstrual cycle.[119] There is no evidence that hormone replacement therapy influences asthma outcome.

Surgery

There are no great problems about surgery in most asthmatics. It is important to remember to use corticosteroids to cover the operation and the early postoperative period if the patient is on long-term oral steroid therapy or has recently stopped it or if the inhaled dose is above 1,600 mcg daily of beclomethasone dipropionate or budesonide. Nebulized bronchodilators can be used for patients on or off ventilators.

Some drugs routinely used during or after anaesthesia may be inappropriate in asthmatic patients. It is of course important to avoid the use of beta blockers. Occasionally asthma can become apparent for the first time when these are used during surgery. Some units use nebulized water from an ultrasonic generator postoperatively to prevent sputum retention. Since hypotonic solutions can provoke bronchoconstriction they should not be used in asthmatics.

Manipulating the airway   Special care is needed in manipulation of the airway. This applies especially to asthmatic patients undergoing bronchoscopy. Atropine is usually used as a premedication to dry secretions and block vagal reflexes. In asthmatic patients the dose should be increased to around 1 mg intravenously or intramuscularly. Ipratropium bromide or beta$_2$ agonists can be given by nebulizer. Particular care must then be taken in anaesthesia of the larynx and airways. Profound laryngospasm or bronchospasm can occur if these precautions are ignored.

Other medical conditions

Thyroid disease   As mentioned in Chapter 3 thyroid disease may interact with the control of asthma. Asthma worsens in hyperthyroidism and usually improves with hypothyroidism.

Nonasthmatic wheezing   Wheezing from localized airway narrowing may sometimes be confused with asthma, but examination and investigations such as the flow volume loop (see Chapter 1) and chest radiograph usually distinguish this.

Widespread wheezing is a feature of the carcinoid syndrome but diarrhoea, facial flushing and hepatomegaly are generally present in addition.

Asthma is usually present for some years as a prelude to allergic granulomatosis (Churg–Strauss syndrome).[120] Evidence for this underlying disorder comes from radiographic changes, evidence of vasculitis and multiorgan disease, raised ESR and high eosinophil count.

Drug sensitivities   A further way in which other medical conditions may be related to asthma is by the limitations the presence of asthma may impose on their treatment. This is mainly a difficulty in a small group of asthmatics who have problems with aspirin and other NSAIDs, for whom alternative analgesics are necessary (see Chapter 3); and with beta blockade in all asthmatics.

No beta blockers presently available are selective enough to be given safely to asthmatics. Fortunately effective alternative drugs are now available for treating angina and hypertension. In hypertension, there is a choice of vasodilators, angiotensin-converting enzyme inhibitors, calcium-channel blockers and other drugs, and in angina, where beta blockers would be chosen, calcium-channel blockers provide the alternative.

Smoking

While we should discourage smoking in all patients, some groups need special attention because adverse effects are more likely. This applies particularly to asthmatics. Many patients find out for themselves that smoking irritates their airways. Although the prevalence of smoking is lower in asthmatics than in the general population, 15–20 per cent continue to smoke.

There are no easy ways of giving up. Patients must be motivated before success is likely. This may come with explanation of the effects of smoke on the airways and the special risks for asthmatics. In general it is easier to convince smokers to stop for an immediate gain, such as improved asthmatic control, rather than a risk of coronary artery disease twenty years in the future. To this end it may help to demonstrate a drop in peak flow rate or an increase in pulse rate on smoking a cigarette. In asthmatics the peak flow will usually drop transiently immediately after one or two deep inhalations from a cigarette.

Once the patient is motivated enough to stop, support is needed to sustain the effort. This comes best from close friends or family and they should be involved in helping if possible. Success rates are better with stopping smoking abruptly, rather than tailing off slowly.

Those patients who, although motivated, have trouble with withdrawal symptoms, may be helped by the use of nicotine patches or chewing gum.[121,122] This is unlikely to help those without a desire to stop or those without symptoms of nicotine withdrawal.

When asthmatics continue to smoke, advice to stop should be reinforced regularly. It is surprising how many such patients say that their doctor never advised them to stop smoking. Cigar and pipe smoke is more irritant than cigarette smoke, and changing the method of smoking tobacco in this way is of little or no benefit.

PRACTICAL POINTS

- Most asthmatics can live a normal life in terms of school, occupational and social life. The practitioner's aim should be to control the condition so that they can do so.
- Only in a small minority do special arrangements need to be made.
- Asthmatics should be encouraged to stay healthy and keep fit, eating sensibly and not smoking.

References

Introduction

1. Ellul-Micallef R, Asthma: a look at the past, *Br J Dis Chest* (1976) **70**: 112–16.

2. Willis T, *Practice of Physick, Pharmaceutice Rationalis or the Operations of Medicine in Humane Bodies* (London 1678).

3. Beasley R, Smith K, Pearse N et al, Trends in asthma mortality in New Zealand, 1908–1986, *Med J Aust* (1990) **152**: 570–3.

4. Hargreave FE, Dolovich J, Newhouse MT, Eds, The assessment and treatment of asthma: A conference report, *J Allergy Clin Immunol* (1990) **85**: 1098–111.

5. Burney P, The epidemiology of asthma, *Allergy* (1993) **48**: 517–21.

6. Citron KM, Pepys J, An investigation of asthma among the Tristan de Cunha islanders, *Br J Dis Chest* (1964) **58**: 119–23.

Chapter 1

7. Corrao WM, Braman SS, Erwin RS, Chronic cough as the sole presenting manifestation of bronchial asthma, *N Engl J Med* (1979) **300**: 633–7.

8. Corris PA, Gibson JG, Asthma presenting as cor pulmonale, *Br Med J* (1984) **288**: 389–90.

9. Empey DW, Laitinen LA, Jacobs L et al, Mechanisms of bronchial hyperreactivity in normal subjects after upper respiratory tract infection, *Am Rev Respir Dis* (1976) **113**: 131–9.

10. Laitinen LA, Laitinen, A, Pathology and cytology of asthma. In: Clark TJH, Godfrey S, Lee TH, eds, *Asthma* (Chapman and Hall: London 1992) 232–53.

11. Rubinfeld AR, Pain MCF, The perception of asthma, *Lancet* (1976) **1**: 882–4.

12. Kikuchi Y, Okabe S, Tamura G et al, Chemosensitivity and perception of dyspnea in patients with a history of near-fatal asthma, *N Engl J Med* (1994) **330**: 1329–34.

13. Prior JG, Cochrane GM, Home monitoring of peak expiratory flow rate using mini-Wright peak flow meter in diagnosis of asthma, *J Roy Soc Med* (1980) **73**: 731–3.

14. Deal EC, McFadden ER, Ingram RH et al, Hyperpnea and heat flux: initial reaction sequence in exercise-induced asthma, *J Appl Physiol* (1979) **46**: 476–83.

15. Webb J, Clark TJH, Chilvers C, Time course of response to prednisolone in chronic airflow obstruction,*Thorax* (1981) **36**: 18–21.

16. Hargreave FE, Ryan G, O'Byrne PM et al, Bronchial responsiveness to histamine in asthma: measurement and clinical significance, *J Allergy Clin Immunol* (1981) **68**: 347–55.

Chapter 2

17. Kelly WJW, Hudson I, Phelan PD et al, Childhood asthma in adult life: a further study at 28 years of age, *Br Med J* (1987) **294**: 1059–62.

18. Speight AWP, Is childhood asthma being underdiagnosed and undertreated? *Br Med J* (1978) **2**: 231–2.

19. Speight AWP, Lee DA, Hey EN, Underdiagnosis and undertreatment of asthma in childhood, *Br Med J* (1983) **286**: 1253–6.

20. McNichol KN, Williams HE, Allon J et al, Spectrum of asthma in children III. Psychological and social components, *Br Med J* (1973) **4**: 16–20.

21. Adinoff AD, Hollester JR, Steroid-induced fractures and bone loss in patients with asthma, *N Engl J Med* (1983) **309**: 265–8.

22. Pearce N, Grainger J, Atkinson M et al, Case-control study of prescribed fenoterol and death from asthma in New Zealand, 1977–81, *Thorax* (1990) **45**: 170–5.

23. Mullen M, Mullen B, Carey M, The association between β-agonist use and death from asthma: a meta-analytic integration of case-control studies, *J Am Med Assoc* (1993) **270**: 1842–5.

24. British Thoracic Association. Death from asthma in two regions of England, *Br Med J* (1982) **285**: 1251–5.

25. Hetzel MR, Clark TJH, Branthwaite MA, Asthma: analysis of sudden deaths and ventilatory arrests in hospital, *Br Med J* (1977) **1**: 808–11.

26. Von Niekerk CH, Weinberg EG, Shore SC et al, Prevalence of asthma: a comparative study of urban and rural Xhosa children, *Clin Allergy* (1979) **9**: 319–24.

27. Sibbald B, Turner-Warwick M, Factors influencing the prevalence of asthma among first degree relatives of extrinsic and intrinsic asthmatics, *Thorax* (1978) 34: 332–7.

28. Cookson WOCM, Young RP, Sandford AJ et al, Maternal inheritance of atopic IgE responsiveness on chromosome 11q, *Lancet* (1992) **340**: 381–4.

29. Atherton DJ, Sewell M, Soothill JF et al, A double-blind controlled crossover trial of an antigen-avoidance diet in atopic eczema, *Lancet* (1978) **1**: 401–3.

30. Brown PJ, Greville HW, Finucane KE, Asthma and irreversible airflow obstruction, *Thorax* (1984) **39**: 131–6.

31. Cockroft DW, Cigarette smoking, airway hyperresponsiveness and asthma, *Chest* (1988) **94**: 675–6.

32. Taylor RG, Gross E, Joyce H et al, Bronchial reactivity and rate of decline in FEV_1 in smokers and ex-smokers, *Thorax* (1983) **38**: 710.

Chapter 3

33. Nicholson KG, Kent J, Ireland DC, Respiratory viruses and exacerbations of asthma in adults, *Br Med J* (1993) **307**: 982–6.

34. Peat JK, van den Berg RH, Green WF et al, Changing prevalence of asthma in Australian children, *Br Med J* (1994) **308**: 1591–6.

35. Platts-Mills TAE, Tovey ER, Mitchell EB et al, Reduction of bronchial hyperreactivity during prolonged allergen avoidance, *Lancet* (1982) **2**: 675–8.

36. Warner JO, Hyposensitization in asthma: a review, *J Roy Soc Med* (1981) **74**: 60–5.

37. Davies RJ, Immunotherapy in respiratory allergy, *Thorax* (1983) **38**: 401–7.

38. Fitch KD, Morton AD, Specificity of exercise in exercise-induced asthma, *Br Med J* (1971) **4**: 577–81.

39. Chilmoncyk BA, Salmun LM, Megathlin KN et al, Association between exposure to environmental tobacco smoke and exacerbations of asthma in children, *N Engl J Med* (1993) **328**: 1665–9.

40. Weitzman M, Gortmaker S, Klein D et al, Maternal smoking and childhood asthma, *Pediatrics* (1993) **85**: 505–11.

41. Anto JM, Horton CE, Rodriguez-Roison R et al, Community outbreaks of asthma associated with inhalation of soybean dust, *N Engl J Med* (1989) **320**: 1097–102.

42. Anto JM, Sunyer J, Reed CE et al, Suitable control measures can eliminate specific air pollution triggers to asthma, *N Engl J Med* (1993) **329**: 1760–3.

43. Tattersfield AE, Beta-blockers in asthma, *Br Med J* (1981) **282**: 901.

44. Cerrina J, Denjean A, Alexandre G et al, Inhibition of exercise induced asthma by a calcium antagonist, nifedipine, *Am Rev Respir Dis* (1981) **123**: 156–60.

45. Patel KR, Sodium cromoglycate and verapamil alone and in combination in exercise induced asthma, *Br Med J* (1983) **286**: 606.

46. Szczeklik A, Gryglewski RJ, Czerniawska-Mysik G, Relationship of inhibition of prostaglandin biosynthensis by analgesics to asthma attacks in aspirin sensitive patients, *Br Med J* (1975) **1**: 67–9.

47. Lunde H, Hedner T, Samuelsson O et al, Dyspnoea, asthma, and bronchospasm in relation to treatment with angiotensin converting enzyme inhibitors, *Br Med J* (1994) **308**: 18–21.

48. Patel KR, Tullet WM, Bronchoconstriction in response to ipratropium bromide, *Br Med J* (1983) **286**: 1318.

49. Lessof MH, Wraith DG, Merrett TG et al, Food allergy and intolerance in 100 patients with local and systemic effects, *Q J Med* (1980) **49**: 259–71.

50. Parkes WR, *Occupational Lung Disorders* (Butterworth: London 1982) 415–53.

51. *Occupational Asthma (Report of Industrial Advisory Council)*, (HMSO: London 1981).

52. Luparello T, Leize N, Lourie CH et al, The interaction of psychological stimuli and pharmacological agents on airway reactivity in asthmatic subjects, *Psychosomatic Med* (1970) **32**: 509–13.

53. Christopher KL, Wood RP, Eckert RC et al, Vocal cord dysfunction presenting as asthma, *N Engl J Med* (1983) **368**: 1566–70.

54. Turner ES, Greenberger PA, Patterson R, Management of the pregnant asthmatic patient, *Annals Intern Med* (1980) **93**: 905–18.

55. Goodall RJR, Eavis JE, Cooper DN et al, Relationships between asthma and gastro-oesophageal reflux, *Thorax* (1981) **36**: 116–21.

Chapter 4

56. Pearson MG, Spence DPS, Ryland I et al, Value of pulsus paradoxus in assessing acute severe asthma, *Br Med J* (1993) **307**: 659.

57. Guidelines on the management of asthma. Statement by the British Thoracic Society et al, *Thorax* (1997) **48** (suppl 1): S1–S24.

58. International consensus report on the diagnosis and management of asthma, *Clin Exp Allergy* (1992) **22** (suppl 1): 1–72.

59. Stewart MF, Barclay J, Warowton R, Risk of giving intravenous aminophylline to acutely ill patients receiving maintenance treatment with theophylline, *Br Med J* (1984) **288**: 450.

Chapter 5

60. Adkinson NF, Eggleston PA, Ehey D et al, A controlled trial of immunotherapy for asthma in allergic children, *N Engl J Med* (1997) **336**: 324–31.

61. Dias PLR, Subramaniam S, Lionel NDW, Effects of acupuncture in bronchial asthma: preliminary communication, *J Roy Soc Med* (1982) **75**: 245–8.

62. Research Committee of the British Tuberculosis Association, Hypnosis for asthma: a controlled trial, *Br Med J* (1968) **4**: 71–6.

63. Hetzel MR, Clark TJH, Comparison of normal and asthmatic circadian rhythms in peak expiratory flow rate, *Thorax* (1980) **35**: 732–8.

64. Ryan G, Latimer KM, Juniper EF et al, Effect of beclomethasone dipropionate on bronchial responsiveness to histamine in controlled non-steroid-dependent asthma, *J Allergy Clin Immunol* (1985) **75**: 25–30.

65. Juniper EF, Kline PA, Vanzieleghem MA et al, Effect of long-term treatment with an inhaled corticosteroid on airway hyperresponsiveness and clinical asthma in nonsteroid-dependent asthmatics, *Am Rev Respir Dis* (1990) **142**: 632–6.

66. Lundgren R, Soderberg M, Horstedt P et al, Morphological studies of bronchial mucosal biopsies from asthmatics before and after ten years of treatment with inhaled steroids, *Eur Respir J* (1988) **1**: 883–9.

67. Woodcock AA, Johnson MA, Geddes DM, Theophylline prescribing, serum concentrations and toxicity, *Lancet* (1983) **2**: 610–12.

68. Sears MR, Taylor DR, Pruit CG et al, Regular inhaled beta-agonist treatment in bronchial asthma, *Lancet* (1990) **336**: 1391–6.

69. Pearlman DS, Chervinsky P, LaForce C et al, A comparison of salmeterol with albuterol in the treatment of mild-to moderate asthma, *N Engl J Med* (1992) **327**: 1420–5.

70. Drazen JM, Israel E, Boushey HA et al, Comparison of regular schedules with as-needed use of albuterol in mild asthma, *N Engl J Med* (1996) **335**: 841–7.

71. James P, Henry J, Cochrane GM, Compliance with therapy in patients with chronic airflow obstruction, *Thorax* (1982) **37**: 778–9.

72. Stokes TC, Morley J, Prospects for an oral Intal, *Br J Dis Chest* (1981) **73**: 1–14.

73. Price JF, Weller PH, Comparison of fluticasone propionate and sodium cromoglycate for the treatment of childhood asthma (an open parallel group study), *Resp Med* (1995) **89**: 363–8.

74. Willey RF, Godden DJ, Carmichael J et al, Comparison of twice daily administration of a new corticosteroid, budesonide,with beclomethasone dipropionate four times daily in the treatment of chronic asthma, *Br J Dis Chest* (1982) **76**: 61–8.

75. O'Byrne PM, Treatment of mild asthma, *Lancet* (1997) **349**: 818.

76. Smith MJ, Hodson ME, High dose beclomethasone inhaler in the treatment of asthma, *Lancet* (1983) **1**: 265–9.

77. Greening AP, Ind PW, Northfield M et al, Salmeterol versus higher-dose corticosteroids in asthma patients with symptoms on existing corticosteroids, *Lancet* (1994) **344**: 219–24.

78. Woolcock A et al, Effect of the addition of salmeterol versus doubling the dose of inhaled steroid in asthmatics, *J Resp Critical Care Med* (1994) **149**: A280.

79. Israel E, Rubin P, Kemp JP et al, The effect of inhibition of 5-lipoxygenase by Zilueton in mild-to-moderate asthma, *Ann Intern Med* (1993) **119**: 1059–66.

80. Britton J, Ayres J, Cochrane GM, Effect of inhaled alpha-blocker on airflow obstruction in asthma, *J Roy Soc Med* (1981) **74**: 646–8.

81. Rudolf M, Riordan JF, Grant BJB et al, Bromhexine in severe asthma, *Br J Dis Chest* (1978) **72**: 307–12.

Chapter 6

82. Bacon CJ, Management of asthma in the child aged under 6 years, *Br Med J* (1981) **283**: 141.

83. Godfrey S, Balfour-Lynn L, Tooley M, A three-to-five year follow-up of the use of the aerosol steroid beclomethasone in childhood asthma, *J Allergy Clin Immunol* (1978) **62**: 335–9.

Chapter 8

84. Lee TH, Brown MJ, Causon R et al, Exercise induced release of histamine and neutrophil chemotactic factors in atopic asthmatics, *J Allergy Clin Immunol* (1982) **70**: 75–81.

85. Morgan DJR, Moodley I, Phillips MJ et al, Plasma histamine in asthmatic and control subjects following exercise: influence of circulating basophils and different assay techniques. *Thorax* (1983) **38**: 771–7.

86. Russell G, Jones SP, Selection of skin tests in childhood asthma, *Br J Dis Chest* (1976) **70**: 104–6.

87. Adkinson NF, The radioallergosorbent test: uses and abuses, *J Allergy Clin Immunol* (1980) **65**: 1–4.

88. Aas K, *The Bronchial Provocation Test* (Charles C Thomas: Springfield, Illinois 1974).

89. Davies RJ, Blainey AD, Evaluation and treatment of house dust mite allergy in perennial rhinitis. In: *Proceedings of the XI International Congress of Allergology and Clinical Immunology* (MacMillan: Basingstoke 1983).

90. Gaddie J, Skinner C, Palmer KN, Hyposensitization with house dust mite vaccine in bronchial asthma, *Br Med J* (1976) 2: 561.

91. Warner JO, Price JF, Soothill JF et al, Controlled trial of hyposensitization to *Dermatophagoides pteronyssinus* in children with asthma, *Lancet* (1978) **2**: 912–15.

92. McAllen MK, Heaf PJD, McInroy P, Depot grass-pollen injections in asthma. Effect of repeated treatment on clinical response and measured bronchial sensitivity, *Br Med J* (1967) **1**: 22–5.

93. Taylor WV, Ohman JL, Lavell FC, Immunotherapy in cat induced asthma. Double blind trial with evaluation of bronchial responses and histamine, *J Allergy Clin Immunol* (1978) **61**: 283–7.

94. Frankland AW, Hughes WH, Gorrell RH, Autogenous bacterial vaccines in the treatment of asthma, *Br Med J* (1955) **2**: 941–4.

95. Glimp RA, Bayer AS, Fungal pneumonias. Part 3, Allergic bronchopulmonary aspergillosis, *Chest* (1981) **80**: 85–94.

96. Safirstein BH, Aspergilloma consequent to allergic bronchopulmonary aspergillosis, *Am Rev Respir Dis* (1983) **108**: 940–3.

97. Lake KB, Browne PM, Van Dyke JJ et al, Fatal disseminated aspergillosis in an asthmatic patient treated with corticosteroids, *Chest* (1983) **83**: 138–9.

Chapter 9

98. Larsson S, Svedmyr N, Bronchodilating effect and side effects of beta$_2$ adrenoceptor stimulants by different modes of administration (tablets, metered aerosol and combination thereof), *Am Rev Respir Dis* (1977) 116: 861–9.

99. Webb J, Rees J, Clark TJH, A comparison of the effects of different methods of administration of beta$_2$-sympathomimetics in patients with asthma, *Br J Dis Chest* (1982) **76**: 351–7.

100. Lillehei JP, Aminophylline oral vs rectal administration, *J Am Med Assoc* (1968) **205**: 530–3.

101. Evans PWG, Craven A, Evans N, Nocturnal wheezing in children: management with controlled release aminophylline, *Br Med J* (1981) **283**: 18.

102. Williams S, Seaton A, Intravenous or inhaled salbutamol in severe acute asthma? *Thorax* (1977) **32**: 555–8.

103. Davies DS, Pharmacokinetics of inhaled substances, *Postgrad Med J* (1973) **51** (suppl 7): 69–75.

104. Connolly CK, Methods of using pressurized aerosols, *Br Med J* (1975) **3**: 21.

105. Newman SP, Pavia D, Clarke SW, How should a pressurized beta-adrenergic bronchodilator be inhaled? *Eur J Respir Dis* (1981) **62**: 3–21.

106. Newman SP, Pavia D, Garland N et al, Effects of various inhalation modes on the deposition of radioactive pressurized aerosols, *Eur J Respir Dis* (1982) **63** (suppl): 57–65.

107. Myers M, Dawkins K, Effect of a timed interval between inhalation of beta-agonist and corticosteroid aerosols on the control of chronic asthma, *Thorax* (1983) **38**: 378–82.

108. O'Callaghan C, Barry P, Spacer devices in the treatment of asthma, *BMJ* (1997) **314**: 1061–2.

109. Rees PJ, Clark TJH, Moren F, The importance of particle size in response to inhaled bronchodilators, *Eur J Respir Dis* (1982) **119** (suppl): 73–8.

110. Clay MM, Pavia D, Newman SP et al, Assessment of jet nebulizers for lung aerosol therapy, *Lancet* (1983) **2**: 592–4.

111. Gunawardena KA, Patel B, Campbell IA et al, Oxygen as a driving gas for nebulizers: safe or dangerous, *Br Med J* (1984) **288**: 272–4.

112. Milner LJR, Crompton GK, Beclomethasone dipropionate and oropharyngeal candidiasis, *Br Med J* (1974) **3**: 797–8.

113. Williams AJ, Baghat MS, Stableforth DE et al, Dysphonia caused by inhaled steroids: recognition of a characteristic laryngeal abnormality, *Thorax* (1983) **38**: 813–21.

Chapter 10

114. Jones DP, O'Conner SA, Collins JV et al, Effects of long term ionised air treatment in patients with bronchial asthma, *Thorax* (1976) **31**: 428–32.

115. Ben-Dov I, Amirav I, Shochina M et al, Effect of negative ionization of inspired air on the response of asthmatic children to exercise and inhaled histamine, *Thorax* (1983) **38**: 584–8.

116. Krenger AP, Andiese PC, Kotaka S, Small air ions: their effect on blood levels of serotonin in terms of modern physical therapy, *Int J Biometerol* (1968) **12**: 225–39.

117. Chu SS, Pearce SJ, Acupuncture point stimulation in bronchial asthma, *Thorax* (1983) **38**: 221–2.

Chapter 11

118. Lindsay D, The benefits of warm-up for asthmatic children. In: Oseid S, Edwards AM, eds, *The Asthmatic Child in Play and Sport* (Pitman: London 1983) 305–10.

119. Harley SP, Asthma variation with menstruation, *Br J Dis Chest* (1981) **75**: 306–8.

120. Edwards CW, Vasculitis and granulomatosis of the respiratory tract, *Thorax* (1982) **37**: 81–7.

121. Jarvis MJ, Raw M, Russell MAH et al, Randomized controlled trial of nicotine chewing gum, *Br Med J* (1982) **285**: 537–40.

122. Tang JL, Law M, Wald N, How effective is nicotine replacement therapy in helping people to stop smoking? *Br Med J* (1994) **308**: 21–6.

Useful addresses

British Lung Foundation
8 Peterborough Mews
London SW6 3BL

British Thoracic Society
1 St Andrew's Place
London NW1 4LB

National Asthma Campaign
Providence House
Providence Place
London N1 0NT

Stratford-upon-Avon Asthma Training Centre
(Director, Greta Barnes)
Winton House
Church Street
Stratford-upon-Avon
Warwickshire
CV37 6HB

Acknowledgements

The publishers are grateful to Terence Carriage for drawing the diagrams; to the Department of Medical Photography, United Medical and Dental Schools of Guy's and St Thomas's Hospitals for the studio photography; to Allen & Hanbury's Limited, Greenford, Middlesex for providing the diary card for use on page 85; and to Judy Chamberlain, Welsh Plant Breeding Station, Aberystwyth, for her help and advice with several of the electron micrographs.

The publishers would like to acknowledge the following individuals and organizations for their assistance with the photographs:
Professor C Mims, Guy's Hospital, London (Fig 1.3, page 6); Gordon Museum, United Medical and Dental Schools of Guy's and St. Thomas's Hospitals (Fig. 1.5, page 8); Sandoz Pharmaceuticals Limited (Fig. 1.6, page 9); SEM Unit, Slough Laboratory, MAFF, Crown copyright (Fig. 3.2, page 29); Dr Jeremy Burgess/Science Photo Library (Figs 3.5 and 3.6, page 31); Heather Angel, Biofotos (Figs 3.3 and 3.4, page 31); Dr Atkey, Glasshouse Crop Research Institute (Fig. 3.8, page 32); Dr Jan Cooper, NERC, Institute of Virology, Oxford (Fig. 3.7, page 32); Professor Tony Newman-Taylor, Brompton Hospital, London (Fig. 3.13, page 42); Ann Dewar, Brompton Hospital, London (Fig. 8.1, page 100); Dr J Reidy, Consultant Radiologist, Guy's Hospital (Fig. 8.8, page 113); Professor Stephen Challacombe and the Department of Dental Illustration, United Medical and Dental Schools of Guy's and St. Thomas's Hospitals (Fig. 9.18, page 137); Racal Group Services Limited (Fig. 11.1, page 146).

Sources
Dodge & Burrows, *Am Rev Respir Dis* (1980) **122**, for Fig. I.1, page x; Clark TJH, Godfrey S, *Asthma*, 1st edn (Chapman and Hall: London 1977) Chapter 3 for Figure 1.14, page 15; Jackson RT, Beaglehole R, Rea HH, Sutherland DC, *Br Med J* (1982) **285**, for Fig. 2.2, page 22; British Thoracic Association, *Br Med J* (1982) **285**, for Fig. 2.3, page 23; Anderson et al, *Br J Dis Chest* (1975) **69**, for Fig. 3.9, page 33; Deal EC, McFaddon ER, Ingram RH, Jaegar JJ, *J Appl Physiol* (1979) **46**, for Fig. 3.10, page 34; Guidelines on the management of asthma. Statement by the British Thoracic Society et al, *Thorax* (1993) **48** (suppl 1), for Fig. 4.7, pages 56–7, Fig. 4.8, pages 58–9, Fig. 5.2, pages 74–5 and Fig. 6.4, pages 88–9; Steenhoek A, Palmen FMHLG, *Respiration* (1984) **45**, for Fig. 9.3, page 118; Webb J, Rees J, Clark TJH, *Br J Dis Chest* (1982) **76**, for Fig. 9.1, page 115; Davies DS, *Postgrad Med J* (1975) **51**(suppl 7), for Fig. 9.4, page 120.

Index

Page numbers in *italics* refer to illustrations

ABPA *see* Allergic bronchopulmonary
    aspergillosis
Acaricides 30
Accolate 71
Accuhaler 69, 86, *128*
ACE inhibitors, action 37
Action plan 60
Acupuncture
    clinical studies 142
    psychological factors 43
Acute (severe) asthma
    assessment of attack 46–51, 56–8
    in childhood *see* Childhood asthma
    ECG 49
    hospitalization 60
    life-threatening
        assessment 56–7
        treatment 58–9
    management 46–61
    outlook 20
    patient education 60
    prevention of attack 51–2
    referral to hospital 94–5
    treatment 52–60
        bronchodilators 52–4
    uncontrolled
        assessment 56–7
        treatment 58–9
    warning signs 50–1
    see also specific aspects
Addresses, useful 156
Administration of drugs *see* Drug delivery
Adrenaline *see* Beta2 agonists
Adrenaline, injected route 119
Aerocom 79
Aerosols
    children 86
    spacers 86

Aetiology, extrinsic vs intrinsic 3
Age at presentation 18
Air ionizers 141–2
Airflow, obstruction
    chronic 25–6
    diagnosis 1–2
    hyperresponsiveness 7
    irreversible 1–2
    masquerading as asthma 43
    tumour 6
Airway, precautions in asthmatics 147
Allergens
    bronchial challenge 109
    hyposensitization therapy 109–11
    purification 110
    radioallergosorbent test (RAST), IgR test 32,
        106–9
    see also specific substances
Allergic bronchopulmonary aspergillosis 44
    diagnosis 111–12, *113*
    treatment 112
Allergic rhinitis 30
    desensitization 110–11
Alpha blockers 77
Alternaria spores 32
Alveolar lavage
    eosinophils 102
    epithelial cells 102
    neutrophils 102
Aminophylline
    acute (severe) asthma 59
    blood levels 117
    factors affecting metabolism 117
    injected route 119
    i.v., acute asthma 53–4
    oral route 116–17
    sensitivity reactions 37
Anaphylactic reactions, penicillin 37
Anaphylaxis, SRSA 102
Angina, treatment 78

Angiotensin-converting enzyme (ACE)
    inhibitors, action 37
Animals 32–3
Antiallergic drugs 77
Antiallergics 77
Antibiotics
    children, contraindications 84, 91
    indications for use 27–8
    precipiating asthma 36
Anticholinergic agents 70–1, 130–2
    see also Ipratropium bromide
Antihistamines 76–7
    children, contraindications 90
Anti-inflammatory drugs 77
Anti-leukotrienes 77, 117
Anxiety 142
Arachidonic acid metabolites 100–2
Aspergillosis, allergic bronchopulmonary,
    diagnosis and treatment 111–13
Aspirin, action 36–7, 148
Assessment, childhood asthma 84
Asthma, definitiobn ix, x
Atenolol, bronchoconstriction 36
Atopy
    children 84
    inheritance of 25
    skin tests 103

Bacterial infections 27–8
Basement membrane, changes 9
Beclomethasone diproprionate
    administration and dosage 68, 136–7
    chronic asthma 76, 79
    growth effects, children 90
    side effects 138
Bed, mattress covers 29
Bee stings 110
Beta2 agonists
    chronic asthma 70
    inhaled route 120–3
    injected route 119
    list and dosage 126
    oral route 114–16
    severe asthma 52–3
    see also specific agonists
Beta blockers
    avoidance 36, 148
    precipitation of asthma 36
Birth order, risk of asthma 25
Blood gases, measurement 50
Bovines, rhinovirus infection 6
Breast feeding 25
Breathing exercises 140
Bronchial challenge 109
    late reactions 109

Bronchial hyperresponsiveness 7
    genetic basis 25
    reduction 66
Bronchial lavage 78, 140–1
Bronchial wall, changes 9
Bronchitis
    chronic, defined 26
    'recurrent' 20
Bronchoconstriction
    inappropriate, produced by asthma
        treatment 37–8
    produced by beta blockers 36
Bronchodilators
    acute asthma 52–4
    increasing need 47, 52–3
    indications 76, 79
    inhaled vs oral 68–9
    nebulizers 70
    new inhalers 69
    powder delivery systems 69
    problems 69
    regular use 68
    severe asthma 52–3
    spacers and extension tubes 70
    see also Salbutamol
Budesonide 76
    administration and dosage 68, 136–7

Calcium channel blockers, indications 36,
    77–8
Candidiasis 135, 137
Carbamazepine, precipitating asthma 36
Cardiovascular effects 48
Cats 32–3
Cattle, rhinovirus infection 6
Challenge testing 16, 17, 42
Chemokines, as target for drug development
    102
Childhood asthma
    assessment 84
    diagnosis 2–3, 80–3
    diary card 85
    growth, effects of corticosteroids 90
    'labelling' 81–2
    management 80–92, 88–9
    morbidity, absence from school 20–1
    outlook 18–20
    overprotection 20–1
    peak flow meters 82, 83
    precipitating factors 83–4
    prognosis 91
    treatment
        acute asthma 87
        antibiotics, contraindications 84, 91
        chronic asthma 87, 88–9, 90
        corticosteroids, effects on growth 90

routes of administration 86–7, 90
side-effects 21–2
summary 91, 92
China, prevalence rate *xi*
Chronic asthma
in childhood *see* Childhood asthma
control
criteria for 62–3
environmental 63–4
management 62–79, *74–5*
treatment
nocturnal asthma 66
prophylaxis 65–6
route of administration 66–7
nocturnal asthma 66
strategy 64–5
Churg–Strauss syndrome 147
Cladosporium spores 32
Climatic change 36
Clinics 93–4
Combined preparations
inhaled 79
oral 78
Combivent 79
Cor pulmonale, diagnosis 2
Corticosteroids
for ABPA 112
acute asthma 54–5
administration 135–8
adrenal suppression 138
BTS recommendations 65
effects on childhood growth 90
inhaled route 73–6, 120–3
oral route 118–19
side-effects 21
trial of, 'run-in period' *16*
Corticosteroids *15*
see also Hydrocortisone; Prednisolone
Cough
in diagnosis 1
presenting symptom 80
Cushing's syndrome 73
Cyclo-oxygenase pathway 101–2
Cyclosporin B 78

Definition of asthma *x*
Dermatographia 105
Dermatophagoides pteronyssinus 29
see also House dust mite
Desensitization (immunotherapy) 63–4
dextrans, contraindications 36
Diagnosis 1–17
childhood asthma 2–3, 80–3
cor pulmonale 2
differential diagnosis 2

paroxysmal nocturnal dyspnoea 2
referral to hospital 94–5
Diary card 85, *96*
Diazepam, avoidance 60
Diet 145
Diskhaler, inhalers 125, *125*
Dogs 32–3
Drugs
drug delivery
inhaled 120–38
injections 119
management 114–39
oral (GI tract) 114–19
dyes, etc., precipitating asthma 36
precipitation of asthma 36–8
regulations, IOC 145
sensitivities in asthmatics 148
in sport 35, 145
Duovent 79
Dyes, in drugs, precipitating asthma 36

ECG, acute asthma 49
Eczema, treatment 77
Education, for patient 60
Education at school 144–5
Emotional factors 42
children 84
Environmental control 63–4
Eosinophils, alveolar lavage 102
Epithelial cells, alveolar lavage 102
Equipment, general practice 95–7
Exercise
general 33–5
recommendations 140
responses *15*
sports 35
warming-up 145
Exercise testing, peal flow 13–15
Exercise-induced asthma
mechanisms 34–5
mimicking 34
nedocromil sodium 33
treatment 77
Extrinsic vs intrinsic aetiology 3

Fenoterol
in combined preparations 79
dosage 126
Flow volume loops *4–5*
Flunisolide 76
Fluticasone propionate, administration and
dosage 76, 136–7
Foods, precipitating factors 38
Formoterol 66
Freeway Lite Luxury Nebulizer/Compressor
system *132*

Gastro-oesophageal reflux 44
Gastrointestinal tract, drug delivery 114–19
General practice
    equipment 95–7
    guidelines for acute severe asthma 56–9
    management 93–8
Gold 78
Grass pollens 30, *31*

H1 blockers, oral, contraindications 76–7
Haemophilus influenzae 28
Histamine testing 16, *17*
Horseness, vocal cord myopathy 135
Hospital doctors, liaison 97–8
Hospitals, referral 94–5
House dust mites 28–30
    acaricides 30
    densensitization 110
Hydrocortisone
    i.v.
        bronchoconstriction 38
        severe asthma 54
    life-threatening asthma 54, 59
    see also Corticosteroids
5-Hydroxytryptamine 142
Hyperresonsiveness, genetics of 25
Hypertension, treatment 78
Hypnosis
    controlled study 142
    psychological factors 43
Hyposensitization
    mites 30
    pollen 30
Hyposensitization therapy, inflammation
    109–11
Hypothalamic function (HPA) 73
Hypoxia, oxygen therapy 55, 59

IgE antibodies
    skin tests 103–9
    speciofic mediators 7
    test, RAST 32
Imidazole, for ABPA 112
Immunological tests 103–9
Immunotherapy 63–4
Industrial Injuries Advisory Council,
    compensation 42
Infections 27–8
Inflammation 99–113
    cellular involvement 99–102
    hyposensitization therapy 109–11
    immunological tests 103–9
    infections 27–8
    neurotransmitters 102, 103
Inhalers
    for children 86

principles of drug delivery 120–38
technique 120–3, *122–3*
types
    Accuhaler 69, 86, *128*
    breath-actuated 124–5
    Diskhaler 125, *125*
    Rotacaps 126
    Spinhaler *133–4*
    Turbohaler 126, *127*
Inheritance of asthma 25
Inheritance of atopy 25
Injections, drug delivery 119
Insect stings 110
Intal 79
Interleukin-5 (IL-5), as target for drug
    development 102
Iodine-based contrast media,
    contraindications 36
Ionizers 141–2
Ipratropium bromide
    action 71
    acute (severe) asthma 59
    administration 130–2
    bronchoconstriction 37
    in combined preparations 79
Itraconazole, for ABPA 112

Ketotifen, anti-inflammatory action 77

Late reactions, bronchial challenge 109
Latent reactions, occupational asthma 40–2, *41*
Leukotriene antagonists 67, 77
5-Lipooxygenase inhibitors 102, 117
Lipoxygenase pathway 100–1
Lung function
    ABA episodes *113*
    deterioration 48
    mucus plugs *8, 9, 141*
    overinflation *48, 49*
    pneumothorax 50
Lymphocytes 102

Macrophages, alveolar lavage 102
Management
    acute asthma 46–61
    bronchoconstriction 37–8
    childhood asthma 80–92
    chronic asthma 62–79
    drug delivery 114–39
    in general practice 93–8
    physiotherapy 140–3
Mast cells *100–1*
Methacholine testing 16, *17*
Methotrexate 78
Methylxanthines, oral route 116–17
Metoprolol, bronchoconstriction 36

Mimicking of asthma 34, *43*
Mineral oil, precipitating asthma 36
Mites *see* House dust mites
Mortality *ix*
  1959–90
    England and Wales *22*
    New Zealand *22*
  1982, deficiencies of assessment 23
Mucolytics 79
Mucus plugs *8, 9*
  in ABPA 112
  bronchial lavage 78, 140–1

Natural history 18–26
Nebulizers 95
  action 129
  bronchodilators 70
  children 86
  Freeway Lite Luxury Nebulizer *132*
  technique 129, *130, 131*
Nedocromil sodium
  action 73
  administration 135
  exercise-induced asthma 33
Neurotransmitters, inflammation 102, 103
Neutrophils, alveolar lavage 102
Nifedipine, indications 77
Nitric oxide 102
Nitrogen dioxide 35
Nocturnal asthma 2, 66, 80
NSAIDs, action 36–7, 148

Occupational asthma 39–42, 145–6
  latent reactions 40–2, *41*
Oral drug delivery 114–19
Osteoporosis 138
Oxitropium bromide
  action 71
  administration 75, 130–2
Oxygen therapy 55
Ozone 35

Paradoxical pulse, measurement *47, 48–9*
Paroxysmal nocturnal dyspnoea,
  diagnosis 2
Pathological changes, factors 8–10
Peak flow
  diary card 11, 85, *96*
  diurnal variation 13, 24
  exercise effects *33*
  exercise testing 13–15
  improvement, with salbutamol 13
  recovery *24*
  and risk 24
  and steroid trial 15–16
  temperature effects *34*

Peak flow meters
  children's use *82, 83*
  measurements *11, 12, 13*
  portable 9–12, *10*
  prescription 97
  use 11–12
Penicillin, anaphylactic reactions 37
Pets 32–3
Physiotherapy, management 140–3
Pirbuterol, dosage 126
Pituitary snuff, precipitating asthma 36
Placebo effect, psychological factors 43
Pneumothorax *50*
Pollens *28*, 30, *31*, 32
  densensitization 110
Pollution 35–6
Precipitating factors 27–45
  childhood asthma 83–4
Prenisolone
  beclomethasone dipropionate equivalent 67
  BTS recommendations 65
  life-threatening asthma 52, 54, 59
  severe asthma 54
  trial of 15, *16*
Prednisolone 15
  see also Corticosteroids
Pregnancy 44, 146–7
Preventative measures 23–4
Prognostic factors 18–20
Provocation of asthma, factors 7, 27–45
Psychological factors 42–3
  children 84
Puberty and menstruation 44, 147
Pulsus paradoxus *47, 48–9*

Radioallergosorbent test (RAST), IgE test 32,
  106–9
Referral, hospitals 94–5
Relaxation techniques 142
Reproterol, dosage 126
Rhinitis, treatment 77
Rhinoviruses 27
  infection, bovine *6*
Rimiterol, dosage 126

Salbutamol
  in combined preparations 79
  in diagnosis 13
  dosage 54, 126
  injected route 119
  oral vs inhaled 67
  severe asthma 52–3
  various routes *115*
Salmeterol, dosage 126
Sedation, avoidance 60
Sex differences 18

Skin tests *103–7*
Sleep disturbance 47
Smoking 26, 35, 148
Socio-economic aspects of asthma 22
Sodium cromoglycate
   administration *133–5*
   bronchoconstriction 37
   children 90
   in combined preparations 79
   introduction 72
   use today 72–3
Sodium dioxide 35
Specific mediators, IgE molecules 7
Spinhaler *133–4*
Spirometry 97
   Vitalograph *14*
Sports 34–5
Steroid trial, and peak flow 15–16
Steroids *see* Corticosteroids
Streptococcus pneumoniae, 28
Sulphasalazine, precipitating asthma 36
Sulphur dioxide, bronchoconstriction 38
Surgery in asthmatics 147
Swimming 34–5

Tachycardia 48
Tartrazine, bronchoconstriction 38
Temazepam, avoidance 60
Terbutaline
   dosage 126
   inhaled route 120–3
   injected route 119
Terfenadine, factors affecting metabolism 77,
   117

Theophylline
   blood levels 117, *118*
   factors affecting metabolism 77, 117
   i.v., acute asthma 53–4
   oral, chronic asthma 67
   oral route 116–17
   problems 71
   therapeutic range *54*
Thyroid disease 44, 147
Timolol, bronchoconstriction 36
Toys 29
Triamcinolone acetonide 76
Tristan da Cunha, prevalence rate *xi*, 25
Turbohaler 126, *127*

Useful addresses 156

Vacuum cleaners, filters 29–30
Ventide 79
Verapamil, indications 77
Virus infections 27–8
Vitalograph, spirometers *14*
Vocal cord myopathy, hoarseness 135

Warfarin, factors affecting metabolism 77,
   117
Wheeze, nonasthmatic 147
Wright's peak flow meter *10*

Yoga 142

Zafirlukast 67, 77, 117
Zilueton 77, 117